Perspectives on the Person with Dementia and Family Caregiving in Ireland

Perspectives on the Person with Dementia and Family Caregiving in Ireland

Suzanne Cahill

Peter Lang
Oxford · Bern · Berlin · Bruxelles · New York · Wien

Bibliographic information published by Die Deutsche Nationalbibliothek
Die Deutsche Nationalbibliothek lists this publication in the Deutsche
Nationalbibliografie; detailed bibliographic data is available on the Internet at
http://dnb.d-nb.de.

A catalogue record for this book is available from the British Library.

Library of Congress Cataloging-in-Publication Data

Names: Cahill, Suzanne, author.
Title: Perspectives on the person with dementia and family caregiving in
   Ireland / Suzanne Cahill.
Description: Oxford ; New York : Peter Lang, [2021] | Includes
   bibliographical references and index.
Identifiers: LCCN 2020042757 (print) | LCCN 2020042758 (ebook) | ISBN
   9781789978513 (paperback) | ISBN 9781800791169 (ebook) | ISBN
   9781800791176 (epub) | ISBN 9781800791183 (mobi)
Subjects: LCSH: Dementia--Patient--Care--Ireland. |
   Dementia--Patients--Family relationships. | Caregivers.
Classification: LCC RC521 .C34 2021 (print) | LCC RC521 (ebook) | DDC
   362.1968/31009415--dc23
LC record available at https://lccn.loc.gov/2020042757
LC ebook record available at https://lccn.loc.gov/2020042758

Cover design by Brian Melville for Peter Lang.

ISBN 978-1-78997-851-3 (print) • eISBN 978-1-80079-116-9 (ePDF)
ISBN 978-1-80079-117-6 (ePub) • ISBN 978-1-80079-118-3 (mobi)

© Peter Lang Group AG 2021

Published by Peter Lang Ltd, International Academic Publishers,
52 St Giles, Oxford, OX1 3LU, United Kingdom
oxford@peterlang.com, www.peterlang.com

Suzanne Cahill has asserted her right under the Copyright, Designs and Patents Act,
1988, to be identified as Author of this Work.

All rights reserved.
All parts of this publication are protected by copyright.
Any utilisation outside the strict limits of the copyright law, without the permission of
the publisher, is forbidden and liable to prosecution.

This applies in particular to reproductions, translations, microfilming, and storage and
processing in electronic retrieval systems.

This publication has been peer reviewed.

I would like to dedicate this book to:
Mná na h'Éireann
In recognition of the valuable and often hidden work many Irish women do as formal and informal caregivers

Contents

Foreword ix

Preface xi

Acknowledgements xiii

Abbreviations xv

CHAPTER 1
An introduction to dementia 1

CHAPTER 2
Models of dementia care 19

CHAPTER 3
Diagnostic and post-diagnostic services 31

CHAPTER 4
The journey to diagnosis and living with dementia: Still me 47

CHAPTER 5
Informal caregivers of people with dementia 57

CHAPTER 6
Personhood, autonomy, capacity and decision-making 75

CHAPTER 7
Long-term residential care					91

CHAPTER 8
Conclusions and future directions				107

References							115

Notes on Contributors						141

Index								143

Foreword

Interest and awareness in dementia in Ireland is high, partly due to the Understand Together Awareness campaign led by the HSE – a programme broadcast on the airwaves and designed to increase understanding, but also because more and more people are affected by dementia either through a family member, friend or work colleague who has been diagnosed. People are finally talking about Alzheimer's disease, and dementia has finally come out of the closet, so to speak.

Despite this heightened awareness many myths still prevail. Some people think that dementia is a normal part of ageing. Many have a huge fear of dementia and believe that a diagnosis is a death sentence. Others think that there is no point in obtaining a diagnosis given that there is no cure for dementia, and several believe that only older people get dementia. In this book Professor Suzanne Cahill attempts to challenge several of these myths by shedding new light on the evidence.

One of the features that make the book appealing is the author's detailed attention to the politics of dementia care and to how these politics have helped to shape the life of the person diagnosed. Throughout the book, the history of how dementia, a condition once neglected and under-resourced in Ireland, finally started to receive political and budgetary attention, is told in a factual, easy-to-absorb way. In this way, it is the only book I know of its kind that brings together in one volume much useful information about dementia and dementia care services in the Irish context.

What is also unique about this book is the way in which boundaries are pushed and an argument is made for the importance of seeing every individual beyond the dementia. So often a person with dementia is regarded as not only having the disease but also being the disease, and in this book the person is placed at the centre stage always.

There are several chapters in the book that particularly appeal to me. One is Chapter 4 where Kathy Ryan, a person like me, who has young-onset dementia, provides a detailed and honest account of her experience of getting a diagnosis and how that diagnosis has impacted on her life. Chapter 6 which addresses the important topics of decision-making, personhood, capacity, autonomy and the new Assisted Decision-Making Capacity Act is both factual and useful. This new Act is complicated and, in the chapter, its components and guiding principles are clearly outlined. It is a sad indictment of Irish society and certainly a key concern of mine that this visionary piece of legislation has still not been fully implemented.

The Irish National Dementia Strategy (2015–2020) will soon expire. This book is timely therefore, given Ireland's ageing population, the increase in prevalence of dementia, the expected decline in the future availability of Irish family caregivers and a national dementia strategy about to come to an end with no impetus for its update or renewal. The book is all the more timely given Covid-19 and the tragic consequences the pandemic has had on the lives of many older Irish people living in nursing homes. Many of those most severely affected by the pandemic have dementia, but sadly they have remained invisible in the entire debate.

It has been a dream for me to work with Professor Suzanne Cahill since my journey through dementia first started in 2012. Her empathy and understanding of the difficulties people like those of us who have this condition experience and her passion for ensuring that our human rights are respected and upheld have been so important for many of us here in Ireland and globally. Her contribution to the field of dementia and ageing both at Trinity College and St James's hospital where she has worked for most of the last two decades has been enormous. This book further consolidates that contribution.

Helen Rochford-Brennan

Preface

There were several reasons behind why I wrote this book. The first is that for years, dementia and especially Alzheimer's disease have been taboo topics in Ireland. Dementia was largely invisible in the health and social care system and hidden from most people. In short dementia was seldom talked about and rarely diagnosed. Then in 2016, the HSE launched a public awareness campaign on dementia. This campaign probably helped many family members open up a conversation about an illness once feared and often associated with guilt, shame and embarrassment. It also created a need for more information on a topic about which no comprehensive Irish book was available. Hence the rationale behind writing this book.

The second reason, which stems from the first, was my hope to bring together in one corpus the wealth of knowledge about dementia that has accumulated in Ireland over a number of decades. For at many levels and in recent times, this new knowledge has been somewhat explosive. It has also been accompanied by a change in public discourse, with a richness in thinking and insights, often led by people who themselves are living with dementia. I wanted to dig deep, collate and analyse information and make it accessible to all those affected by dementia at the coalface. I also wanted to make it accessible to the public and to all those that are very hard working in the field of dementia care in Ireland.

The third reason relates to whom this book is dedicated – *Mná na h'Éireann*. Dementia is clearly a gendered issue: more women than men develop dementia and many more women than men are involved in care roles, both as formal and informal caregivers. These are women whose unpaid or poorly paid work behind closed doors often goes unnoticed. They are women who need a lot more support and recognition for the wide range of health and social care services they deliver, often at enormous personal sacrifice. Therefore, throughout the chapters an appeal is made for more government support for formal and informal caregivers.

This book is a bit of a smörgåsbord. It straddles many different areas but its key storyline, and one that I hope I have made clear, is that all of us must work hard to see the *person* beyond the *dementia* and to preserve that person's dignity, humanity and selfhood, since how the person is regarded and treated will significantly affect their quality of life. The complexities and challenge of dementia mean that it requires multiple responses drawing on multiple frameworks and we need to work collaboratively and not in silos.

Finally, as shown throughout the chapters of this book, the dementia landscape has changed significantly and for the better in Ireland over recent years and we are now at a critical juncture. To complete this process of change, further effort is needed in these most testing of times. I hope this book will add fuel to the movement currently underway in Ireland to improve how the person with dementia is understood, supported and treated by others.

Acknowledgements

There are many people who have supported me while writing this book. Several are colleagues who have influenced me during the years I worked at St James's hospital and at Trinity College Dublin, but there are also other more distant friends and colleagues, who in the past have patiently mentored me. In this context I want to thank Professor Margaret Shapiro at the University of Queensland in Australia. It is difficult to overstate the influence Margaret has had on my career and life.

More locally a number of friends and colleagues have read and provided helpful feedback on different chapters of this book and for this I am most grateful. They include Professor Eamon O'Shea, Dr Maria Pierce, Dr Sarah Donnelly, Dr Niamh Hennelly, Dr Ana Diaz-Ponce, Dr Tony Foley, Dr Dianne Gove and Professor Steve Zarit. Your insights have greatly enriched these chapters. In recent years, I have been privileged to get to know Professor Steve Sabat and I am grateful to Steve for the significant guidance he has given me on topics of mutual concern. Daphne Stevenson and Suzy Cox are both very close friends and social work colleagues of mine. They have tirelessly read and edited each and every chapter of this book and have provided me with their rich insights. I cannot thank either of them enough for their kind support and for always keeping me on track.

A big thank you to Kathy Ryan whose powerful chapter based on her own life experience with dementia has greatly enriched this book. Kathy's honesty and willingness to share her experiences will no doubt help other people living with dementia and their caregivers.

The librarians at Trinity College never cease to amaze me and a big shout out to each of you for your endless support day and night, and to my colleagues in the School of Social Work and Social Policy, a big thank you to all of you there.

At the Institute of Gerontology in Jönköping University, I would like to thank Dr Linda Johansson, Dr Maria Ernsth-Bravell and Susanne

Johannesson for your kindness and especially for waiting for me. You know what I mean!

This book is long overdue and I am most grateful to Anthony Mason, commissioning editor from Peter Lang, for his confidence in me and patience. You have been a pleasure to work with.

Finally, I would like to thank my family in Ireland especially my sisters Jackie and Michele and their families and to my family in Sweden, especially Rigmor and Olle, who have kindly allowed me to use the picture taken of them at Powerscourt in Wicklow for the book's front cover. From the beginning to the end of this project, my husband Thomas has been unbelievable: his love, enthusiasm, encouragement and practical help, including major technical support especially when this computer literally crashed, have been nothing less than astounding. Utan dig skulle detta inte ha kunnat slutföras, du är en på miljonen!

Abbreviations

A&N:	Australian and New Zealand Society for Geriatric Medicine
AD dementia:	Alzheimer's disease dementia, the most advanced of three phases of dementia described in this new model
ADI:	Alzheimer's Disease International
ADM:	Assistant-Decision-Maker
ADMCA:	Assisted Decision-Making Capacity Act
AE:	Alzheimer Europe
ASI:	Alzheimer Society of Ireland
CDM:	Co-Decision-Maker
CR:	Cognitive Rehabilitation
CRPD:	UN Convention on the Rights of Persons with Disabilities
CSF:	Cerebrospinal Fluid
CSO:	Central Statistics Office
CST:	Cognitive Stimulation Therapy
DAI:	Dementia Alliance International
De-Stress:	A study to assess the health and well-being of spousal carers of people with dementia in Ireland
DMR:	Decision-Making Representative
DOH:	Department of Health
DSIDC:	Dementia Services Information and Development Centre
DXA:	Bone Densitometry Scan
ECAD:	Enhancing Care in Alzheimer's Disease
EDJN:	European Data Journalism Network
EEG:	Electroencephalogram

EPA:	Enduring Power of Attorney
GP:	General Practitioner
HCR:	Health Care Representative
HIQA:	Health Information Quality Authority
HCPS:	Home Care Packages
HSE:	Health Service Executive
IHCP:	Intensive Home Care Packages
MCI:	Mild Cognitive Impairment
NDO:	National Dementia Office
NDS:	National Dementia Strategy
NHR:	Nursing Home Regulations
NHSS:	Nursing Home Support Scheme Act
NICE:	National Institute for Clinical Excellence
NTPF:	National Treatment and Purchase Fund
OECD:	Organisation for Economic Co-operation and Development
PEI:	Psychosocial Educational Interventions
PREPARED:	Primary Care Education Pathways and Research in Dementia
SCIE:	Social Care Institute for Excellence, London
SNDS:	Scotland's National Dementia Strategy
UCC:	University College Cork, Ireland
WHO:	World Health Organization

CHAPTER 1

An introduction to dementia

Introduction

The magnitude of dementia cannot be under-estimated. All of us know someone who has dementia or who has been directly or indirectly affected by it, but public knowledge and understanding varies and there is confusion about what dementia is and what it is not. There is also confusion about Alzheimer's disease: the difference between *Alzheimer's disease* and *dementia* and more recently the difference between *Alzheimer's disease* and *Alzheimer's disease dementia* (AD dementia).

The purpose of this chapter is twofold. First it introduces the reader to dementia – an umbrella term used to refer to a group of symptoms affecting memory, thinking and social abilities and to Alzheimer's disease – a specific dementia sub-type. In doing so, it details what these conditions are and what they are not. There are several hundred different types of dementia and the first part of the chapter briefly reviews four of the most frequently occurring sub-types: their symptoms, prevalence rates, risk factors (modifiable and non-modifiable) and lifestyle habits that may help avoid or delay the onset of dementia symptoms. The second part of the chapter progresses to a brief overview of dementia in Ireland to set the context for the chapters to follow. Recent updated estimates are provided on Irish incidence and prevalence rates of dementia and an overview is presented on the political context underpinning the development of Irish health and social care policy in the field of dementia care.

What is dementia?

Dementia is a general clinical term used to describe a group of disorders that have common symptoms but different causes. These symptoms include impairments in memory, orientation, understanding, judgment, calculation, learning, language and thinking (Luengo-Fernandez et al., 2010). However, to constitute dementia, these impairments must be of sufficient severity to interfere with social or occupational functioning (Stephan and Brayne, 2010). A diverse range of conditions cause dementia, but Alzheimer's disease is by far the most common dementia subtype accounting for between 50% to 70% of all dementia cases (Winblad et al., 2016).

Age is the single strongest risk factor for dementia, but dementia is not a natural or inevitable consequence of ageing (WHO, 2019) and a small minority of people aged less than 65 years will also develop the condition (Rossor et al., 2010). The most common early symptoms of dementia include short-term memory loss but as dementia progresses a wide range of other symptoms including disorientation, mood swings, behavioural changes, language deficits and mobility difficulties will arise. Only 20% to 50% of people who have dementia will ever have a documented diagnosis, and probably substantially fewer people living in low to middle income countries will have a diagnosis (Winblad et al., 2016).

Dementia is a progressive and generally irreversible condition: this means that symptoms cannot usually be halted and the impact the condition has on the person's physical, cognitive, behavioural and social functioning will progress over time. This progression varies; some people will have similar general symptoms but the degree to which the symptoms will affect the individual will be different (NICE, 2018) and may be complicated by other often age-related health conditions and/or sensory impairments. Dementia has been described in terms of stages (Winblad et al., 2016) – early (mild), middle (moderate) and late (severe). Although this staging classification exists, it is not always that helpful (Kitwood, 1997a), as not every person diagnosed will experience the progression of symptoms in the same manner.

An introduction to dementia

Dementia is a seriously disabling condition and its progressive nature means that over time, the person will experience deterioration in multiple cognitive domains. Once diagnosed, a person may live three to nine years on average and in some cases up to twenty years (Winblad et al., 2016) but to live well and have a good quality of life, especially in the later stages, the person will need support from a well-trained workforce and from family and friends who can respond to their complex and multiple needs.

Apart from being progressive, dementia is also a chronic life-threatening disability, where the individual may ultimately benefit from palliative care services. No cure or effective treatments are currently available to relieve the symptoms of dementia; available pharmaceutical and psychosocial treatments and interventions are not disease-modifying and can only improve some of the symptoms and only in some of the people affected. This is despite the fact that new drug therapies and psychosocial interventions are being continuously investigated. Clinical trials are at various stages of progress as is the testing of psychosocial interventions. Attempting to consolidate findings from both clinical trials and psychosocial interventions has also been a recent development (Vernooij-Dassen et al., 2019).

The scale of dementia globally and in Europe

The scale of dementia is huge. Globally about fifty million people have the condition and of these, close to ten million are estimated to live in Europe (AE, 2019). There are also about ten million new cases of dementia arising worldwide every year (WHO, 2019). Population ageing means that in the absence of a cure, the numbers of people with dementia will reach 131 million by 2050. The greatest increase in prevalence rates will occur in low to middle income countries (Winblad et al., 2016) as this is where population ageing is occurring most rapidly (WHO, 2012).

Dementia is indiscriminate in whom it targets. It affects men and women, rich and poor, young and old and its economic impact is also enormous. In 2018, the global cost of dementia was estimated to reach US $1 trillion (ADI, 2015). In fact, if it were a country, dementia would represent the 18th largest economy in the world (ADI, 2015). Although care for people living with dementia is provided by several different sectors, social care and informal care account for the greatest costs of dementia care and exceed those costs associated with medical care (WHO, 2012). Globally the challenge of dementia is enormous, and it is little wonder that worldwide, governments are being encouraged to develop policy plans for dementia (OECD, 2015; WHO, 2012, 2017) to help reduce the economic social and emotional costs the condition poses.

There are a myriad of different diseases and conditions that cause dementia of which by far the most common is Alzheimer's disease (Reves et al., 2018). Other common dementias are: vascular dementia, mixed dementia (a combination of Alzheimer's disease and vascular dementia), dementia with Lewy bodies and frontotemporal dementia (Winblad et al., 2016). The section to follow will briefly describe four of these most common dementia sub-types starting with a particular focus on Alzheimer's disease.

Alzheimer's disease: Changes in understandings

Alzheimer's disease was first called after a Bavarian Psychiatrist and Neurologist who in 1907 diagnosed a woman aged 51 with young-onset dementia (Alzheimer, 1907). She presented to him with a severe cognitive disorder. Her symptoms included impaired language, delusions, memory loss and hallucinations (seeing people or objects absent in reality and/or hearing voices also absent). Historically Alzheimer's disease was considered a pre-senile or young-onset type of dementia (Vernooij-Dassen et al., 2019). It was by definition a rare disease affecting people generally aged between 45 and 65 years.

It was not until the late 1960s that a group of US scientists discovered that the brains of older people who died with late-onset dementia, then called senility (Kahn, 1975), had the exact same features of Alzheimer's disease previously believed to be unique to young people (Blessed et al., 1968). This finding led to the elimination of age as a criterion for Alzheimer's disease. It also spawned the development of an Alzheimer's disease movement worldwide and led to the disease pathology or biomedical model of dementia where the race to find a cause, cure and effective treatments commenced. This shift in understanding of Alzheimer's disease also led to some confusion as until then, most people understood Alzheimer's disease to mean early senility or young-onset dementia.

A further factor leading to confusion about the meaning of Alzheimer's disease is the new language first proposed about a decade ago (Dubois et al., 2010; Giaccone et al., 2011) and now used to refer to Alzheimer's disease (Jack Jr et al., 2018). The current and new definition of Alzheimer's disease encompasses the full spectrum of the disease. This includes: (i) *the preclinical stages of Alzheimer's disease* where an abnormal build-up of a protein called amyloid exists – the hallmark of Alzheimer's disease – but the person does not experience any symptoms to (ii) *mild cognitive impairment (MCI) due to Alzheimer's disease* and also referred to *as prodromal AD* where very mild symptoms are in evidence as well as (iii) *the dementia phase* where symptoms are severe enough to impact on daily life. In this new disease model, Alzheimer's disease is understood as a continuum and Alzheimer's disease dementia (AD dementia) is the most advanced of the three phases described in this continuum (AE, 2016). This changing definition of Alzheimer's disease and changing use of existing terms has happened as a result of biomedical research carried out by eminent clinicians and researchers in the field: research that is ongoing (AE, 2016). In this new classification, *Alzheimer's disease is a disease process* in the brain that can but does not always lead to AD dementia. However, AD dementia occurs when there is evidence of cognitive symptoms or deficits which impact on how a person can function in their daily life. Its physiopathology typically includes abnormal build-up of amyloid (plaques) and tau (proteins) in the brain.

According to Jefferies and Agrawal (2009), the typical characteristics of AD dementia (what they classified as Alzheimer's disease) are of progressive day-to-day memory loss problems, visuospatial and perceptual deficits but well-preserved language and social functioning[1]. AD dementia is more

---

1   One must also keep in mind the fact that dementia is also a disability and the apparent symptoms and difficulties experienced are not always solely linked to the biomedical pathology.

common in women than men and prevalence rates increase with age. The average duration of the illness is eight years (Jefferies and Agrawal, 2009).

Other dementia sub-types

In vascular dementia, the second most common dementia sub-type, caused by either a partial or a more permanent cut-off of blood supply to the brain, symptoms may be more abrupt and may include difficulties with problem-solving, delay in thinking and in focus. These symptoms may be more noticeable than memory loss. This dementia sub-type is often characterized by a step-wise progression and sudden episodes of decline. In addition, poor concentration and communication and physical symptoms such as paralysis or limb weaknesses may also be present (Stephan and Brayne, 2010).

In dementia with Lewy bodies, considered by some to be the third most common sub-type and where small clumps of protein build up inside nerve cells, the illness is characterized by progressive cognitive decline, fluctuating cognition, the presence of Parkinsonian symptoms and visual hallucinations that are typically detailed, recurrent and well formed (Jefferies and Agrawal, 2009).

Frontotemporal dementia accounts for fewer than 5% of all dementias, but tends to be more prevalent in younger people. The hallmark of this sub-type is: the early alteration in personality and social conduct (behaviour), with relative intact memory, perception and visuospatial skills (Jefferies and Agrawal, 2009). Although presentations of this dementia sub-type are variable, frontotemporal dementia is also often characterized by reduced motivation, reduced empathy, impaired planning and judgement skills and language and speech problems (Jefferies and Agrawal, 2009). So, a person previously reserved may, because of frontotemporal dementia, become extrovert, blunt in their social interactions and disinhibited. This is behaviour that may cause family members embarrassment and distress.

As mentioned earlier, a small proportion of people aged less than 65 will develop a rare form of dementia commonly known as young-onset dementia (Kelley et al., 2008; Koopmans and Rosness, 2014). This form of dementia accounts for about 5% of all cases (Winblad et al., 2016). Also called *working age dementia*, young-onset dementia poses unique challenges, since often the person has dependent children, may still be gainfully employed and have significant financial commitments including a mortgage. Apart from the financial costs associated, the emotional, psychological and social costs are also very considerable (Hayo et al., 2018). Children may react strongly to a parent's changed behaviour: they may feel embarrassed, ashamed and experience a sense of abandonment. Sadly, some children may be required to take on caregiving roles (Hutchinson et al., 2016). Spouses may have to juggle parenting and caregiving roles or take up employment due to financial hardship. People with an intellectual disability such as Down's syndrome are also at heightened risk of developing young-onset dementia as a result of their carrying extra copies of chromosome 21.

Risk factors for Alzheimer's disease

Different risk factors – like age, gender and genes and broadly speaking non-modifiable, (meaning they can never be changed) and other risk factors like lifestyle and behaviour and potentially modifiable, (meaning they can be changed) are said to contribute to dementia. In terms of non-modifiable risk factors, age is by far the strongest risk factor for Alzheimer's Disease with one in fourteen people over the age of 65 and one in six people over the age of 80 likely to develop the condition (Prince at al., 2014). This is why countries witnessing population ageing including low to middle income countries are concerned about current and future increases in prevalence of Alzheimer's disease (ADI, 2015; Winblad et al., 2016). We also know that women run a slightly higher risk of developing Alzheimer's disease although the exact reasons for this are not well understood and may be related to pathogenetic mechanisms (Viña and Lloret, 2010).

In terms of modifiable risk factors, increasingly we know a lot more about the role cigarette smoking, high blood pressure, obesity, high cholesterol, diabetes, lack of physical exercise and excess alcohol consumption play in contributing to dementia (Winblad et al., 2016; WHO, 2019). We know, for example, that about 30% to 40% of all dementia is preventable (Livingston et al., 2017; 2020) and that about 11% is attributable to cardiovascular risk factors, (Livingston et al., 2020). We know too that brain health, including enjoying a healthy lifestyle in early to mid-life along with protecting our heads (avoiding serious brain trauma that causes unconsciousness) can help to reduce the risk of developing dementia in later life (Shively et al., 2012; Winblad, 2016). We know that a Mediterranean diet (one rich in fruit, vegetables, whole grain, nuts, beans, berries and fish especially oily fish, such as mackerel and salmon) can be very beneficial for our brain health (National Institute on Ageing). We also know that physical exercise along with cognitive stimulation – keeping our brains challenged and stimulated, as well as enjoying novel experiences and remaining socially engaged helps to build new connections between our brain cells and helps to build up cognitive reserve (Pertl et al., 2017).

Cognitive reserve

A relatively new discovery is the concept of *cognitive reserve*, a term used to refer to the: 'mismatch between the degree of age or disease–related neural pathology and the clinical manifestation of that pathology' (Pertl et al., 2017, p. 2). The cognitive reserve hypothesis proposes that enriching experiences can change the structure and function of the brain to the extent that some people can withstand greater brain damage before showing symptoms of cognitive dysfunction (Stern, 2009). Social factors including novel experiences and engagement in mentally stimulating leisure-time activities can influence brain structure and may contribute to cognitive reserve (Fratiglioni and Wang, 2007). It has been argued that by building up cognitive reserve we may be able to delay the possibility of presenting with symptoms of dementia (Stern, 2009).

What is not dementia

Whilst most dementias are progressive and irreversible, a small number of conditions mimic dementia and when identified can be fully reversed (Bello and Schultz, 2011). These conditions include thyroid and vitamin deficiencies, chronic stress, brain tumours, severe depression, delirium and chronic fatigue. Excessive alcohol consumption leading to Korsakoff's disease – an alcohol induced dementia where toxins from alcohol essentially poison brain cells – is also reversible depending on its severity and on what stage in the course of the disease a person decides to stop drinking alcohol.

The interactions of certain medications, often taken by older people to treat other health conditions can sometimes produce dementia-like symptoms. This is why a person who is worried about their memory or cognitive decline should always obtain a medical assessment and diagnosis. A minority of people also worry about their memory but on assessment have no pathology or underlying memory or cognitive problems. This group of people are often referred to as *subjective memory complainers* or *the worried well*.

Many older people also experience memory lapses, sometimes glibly referred to as senior moments. It is not uncommon for those who experience these lapses to worry they are developing dementia. Have you ever bumped into someone you have not seen for years and are unable to remember their name, or gone upstairs to find something and then forgotten what you were looking for? As we age, a little forgetfulness, often referred to as *age-related memory problems*, is not uncommon. However if the forgetfulness is severe enough to interfere with the ability to carry out one's normal daily life, then a more sinister problem may be developing. Also contrary to what was once popular belief, severe memory loss once known as *advanced senility* is not a normal or typical part of growing older.

Mild cognitive impairment

Mild cognitive impairment (MCI) can be defined as cognitive decline greater than that expected for a person's age and education but where the decline does not interfere significantly with a person's ability to undertake activities of daily living (Lawlor and Brennan, 2016). In other words, it is where symptoms of memory loss or cognitive decline are identified through various assessment tests, but these symptoms do not adversely affect everyday life. There are different kinds of MCI. For example, MCI due to Alzheimer's disease also known as prodromal AD (Jack Jr et al., 2011; McKhann et al., 2011) is a specific type of MCI that almost probably leads to AD dementia but the progression from MCI in general to dementia is not as certain.

Treatments for Alzheimer's disease

The early 1990's saw the introduction of the first drug developed to treat dementia (Banerjee, 2015) and there are currently four drugs on the market for the treatment of Alzheimer's disease, three of which are cholinesterase inhibitors and the other is memantine. Commonly referred to as anti-dementia drugs, these drugs are based on the cholinergic hypothesis[2] and none are considered disease-modifying, meaning they cannot alter the underlying problem causing the disease. In the case of Alzheimer's disease, cholinesterase *inhibitors* (called so because they are said to *inhibit* the breakdown of *acetylcholine*, a chemical and neurotransmitter required for our brains to work efficiently) are generally prescribed for mild to moderate stages; and memantine is often prescribed for severe

---

2   The cholinergic hypothesis now over twenty years old suggests that the depletion of a chemical found in the brain called acetylcholine and required for our memory to work efficiently contributes to cognitive decline in older people with Alzheimer's dementia.

stages. Drugs work in about one third of cases and can help with some symptoms for a period of time.

Many of the drugs trialled in recent years for Alzheimer's disease have attempted to diminish the accumulation of beta amyloid in the brains of people with either MCI or who have very mild stages of dementia in the hope that these drugs can halt the progression of the disease and prevent AD dementia. However, to date several of the trials have failed. In 2019, a pharmaceutical company called Biogen announced that one of their phase three drug trials, discontinued earlier that year following the results of a futility analysis, had now obtained positive results following the analysis of data obtained from an additional sample of people. The drug is currently with the Federal Drug Administration. To date, it remains to be seen if this drug will be approved and will come to the market in its current format or whether further research will be required (Bradshaw, 2020). Accordingly, as drug trials targeting beta amyloid fail, researchers are also moving forward in an attempt to combine several different treatment approaches for inflammation, metabolic dysfunction, epigenetic changes and so on.

So far, this chapter has provided broad insights into dementia, a term used to describe a group of disorders that have common symptoms but different causes. It has also discussed some of the most common types of dementia namely Alzheimer's disease, vascular dementia, dementia with Lewy bodies and frontotemporal dementia and has provided a brief overview of treatments. But given that this book is about dementia in Ireland, the second part of this chapter will now advance to a brief discussion about dementia in an Irish policy context, commencing with an overview of population ageing in Ireland and the expected increase in prevalence and incidence rates of dementia.

Dementia in Ireland

Compared with other European countries, like Sweden, Italy, Germany and France, Ireland still has a relatively young population (Eurostat, 2018). In the 2016 Irish Census, there were 637,567 Irish people aged 65 and over, representing 13.4% of the population (CSO, 2016). Depending on what method is used for calculation, that figure could increase to 1.6 million by 2051 (CSO, 2017) representing between 23% and 27% of the total population. A close analysis of population projections, reveals that the *old-old* or those aged over 80 years, is set to rise even more significantly by 2051, increasing in numbers from 147,800 in 2016 to 549,000 (CSO, 2017). These population projections are important, as the *old-old* are that cohort at an exceptionally heightened risk of developing dementia. Accordingly, unless a cure is found in the foreseeable future, Ireland will witness a very significant increase in the numbers of people presenting with dementia.

To prepare for the challenge of dementia, in 2014, the country launched its first national dementia strategy (NDS), a policy plan providing a five-year roadmap for the development and expansion of dementia services (DOH, 2014). Although always signalled as cost neutral, once launched, the Strategy secured funding of over €30 million. This was matched funding obtained from the Atlantic Philanthropies and the HSE (O'Shea and Carney, 2017). A year after its launch, a National Dementia Office (NDO) was established, staffed by a small number of health service professionals whose remit was to implement this policy plan.

Incidence and prevalence rates of dementia in Ireland

To guide the development of the NDS, incidence and prevalence rates of dementia in Ireland were generated in 2012 (Cahill et al., 2012) and updated in 2014, (see Pierce et al., 2014). However, for further planning purposes and using three different methodologies, new prevalence and incidence rates have more recently been generated (Pierse et al., 2019). Based on the 2016 Census, these new prevalence rates suggest that there are between 39,272 and 55,266 Irish people likely to have dementia. Over the next thirty years, these prevalence rates are expected to increase at an average rate of 3.6% per year. This means that by 2036, prevalence rates will have doubled to 115,426 and by 2046 to have almost trebled to 157,883 (O'Shea et al., 2019). Pierse et al.'s work (2019) has also shown that there are currently between 7,752 and 13,733 new cases of dementia in Ireland every year. There are also between 2,906 and 4,311 people in Ireland with young-onset dementia (Pierse et al., 2019). These estimates are important as they remind us of the scale of dementia in Ireland and enable policy makers to plan for the future.

Irish government policy

Like other countries around the world, the stated objective of government policy in Ireland has always been to keep older people including those who have dementia, living in their homes for as long as possible (DOH, 2014) and this is what people with dementia themselves desire (Keogh et al., 2019). It is no surprise, therefore, that about two thirds of all Irish people who have dementia live at home in the community, supported by family members (see Chapter 5) and *if lucky* by government services. The current demand for home care services outweighs supply: wait listing is generally long and the Home Support Service Scheme is considered weak and under-developed (O'Shea et al., 2019). Home care services are extremely variable with a postcode lottery system in evidence. No legislation exists in Ireland today entitling frail older people including those with dementia to home-based community care services, although during 2020, the government had intended to trial a statutory universal home care scheme (The Institute of Public Health, 2017; O'Shea et al., 2019). Due to Covid-19 however, this project appears to have been put on hold.

In 2015, as part of the roll out of the NDS, a large component of the ring-fenced funding allocated to dementia, about €20.5 million was assigned to the delivery and evaluation of intensive home care packages (IHCP) for people diagnosed with dementia with high dependency needs (Keogh et al., 2018a). The programme showed that investment in IHCP helped to keep people at home for longer, even those with significant levels of disability and cognitive impairment.

Whilst the NDS prioritized care in the community, limited attention was given to long-term residential care where about one third of all Irish people who have dementia live. Most of these people live in large-scale generic nursing homes not customized for their complex and unique needs. There are few alternatives to the nursing home model for Irish people who can no longer live at home because of dementia (O'Shea et al., 2019). This is despite repeated calls for a broader range of long-term care options to be made available (Cahill et al., 2014; O'Shea et al., 2019). Chapter 7 in this book will address this topic in greater detail.

Understandings of dementia

Many myths and misunderstandings about dementia prevail in Ireland and like in other countries there is a widespread lack of understanding of causes, symptoms, treatments and prognosis (Cahill et al., 2015b). As part of the NDS, a small but not insignificant proportion of funding, €3 million, was allocated to deliver and evaluate a public awareness programme on dementia[3] (<www.understandtogether.ie>). As part of this campaign, a national survey was first conducted to obtain baseline data about the public's understanding of the condition. Findings demonstrated there was an urgent need to educate Irish people about dementia (Glynn et al., 2017). For example, only 39% of people surveyed were confident that they knew the difference between normal ageing and dementia. Knowledge of risk factors and protective factors for dementia was extremely low and a large proportion of those surveyed were not aware that young people can get dementia. Reflecting the stigma of dementia in Irish society, about one third of respondents reported that if they had dementia, they would not tell their friends or family.

---

3   Understand Together is a public awareness, support and information initiative led by the HSE and delivered in partnership with the ASI and Genio. Launched in 2016, the campaign was designed to increase public awareness and understanding of dementia and create more inclusive and dementia-friendly communities (De Siún and Guiry, 2018).

These findings are not surprising as for years in Ireland, dementia has remained hidden, seldom talked about and rarely diagnosed. More recently a number of valuable community initiatives, too numerous to detail here, have been launched to help people to live well with dementia, participate in everyday life and remain socially engaged. Initiatives such as these have arisen as a result of efforts by the Irish Working Group on dementia (a self-advocacy group), the Alzheimer Society of Ireland (ASI) and the work of organizations committed to best practice, like the Dementia Services Information and Development Centre [DSIDC] (<www.dementia.ie>). Work programmes and initiatives like these, along with many others emerging in Ireland, foster collaboration between local community organizations and encourage the development of dementia inclusive approaches that contribute to a more supportive society for all.

Cost of dementia

In Ireland the cost of dementia is estimated to be over €1.69 billion per annum with the average cost per person estimated to be €35,000. Just under half (48%) of all costs are attributed to the opportunity costs of informal caregivers (Connolly et al., 2014). In 2010, family and friends delivered an estimated 81 million hours of care to people with dementia, saving the Irish government an estimated €807 million. Irish people believe that the care of older citizens is essentially a family responsibility (Citizens' Assembly, 2017) and although informal caregivers want to care, they also want recognition from the State for the very significant contribution they make (O'Shea, 2003). A further 43% of all costs of dementia care in Ireland are accounted for by residential long-stay care, while formal health and social care services such as respite, meals on wheels and home help contribute only 9% to the total costs of dementia. The impact dementia has on the acute health care system in Ireland has also recently been acknowledged. One study has shown that the extended length of stay in hospitals for people diagnosed with dementia costs the government close to €200 million per annum (Connolly and O'Shea, 2015).

Role of the Atlantic Philanthropies

Before concluding this opening chapter, acknowledgement must be given to the substantial contribution the Atlantic Philanthropies has made to dementia care in Ireland for more than a decade[4]. Earlier, reference was made to the role Atlantic played, in financing the implementation of the NDS in 2014. However, this was not a once off commitment – rather Atlantic's investment programme in dementia in Ireland had commenced in 2005[5] and since then has expanded significantly. In funding, for example, the research review underpinning the NDS, (Cahill et al., 2012) along with a myriad of other dementia-related policy, practice and research initiatives, straddling every stage of the dementia journey from diagnosis to end of life, Atlantic has acted as a catalyst, driving much needed change in Irish government policy on dementia. Its significant investment programme (funding a total of fifteen different dementia projects) has drawn attention to an area previously under-funded and under-prioritized and has helped to positively shape the experience of dementia in Ireland. Atlantic's total investment of over €33 million in dementia programmes, has leveraged an additional €51 million from several sources especially government. In so doing Atlantic has served to widen and deepen capacity and leadership in dementia care in Ireland. In short Atlantic's investment programme has transformed the dementia care landscape in Ireland.

Conclusions

This chapter has introduced the reader to dementia, describing what the condition is what it is not. It has also outlined the scale of dementia is in Ireland, in Europe and globally. There are many different types of

---

4   For a full comprehensive overview of Atlantic's investment in dementia services in Ireland see: *Dementia Paying Dividends* (O'Shea and Carney, 2017).
5   Atlantic's preliminary discussions commenced with the DSIDC in 2005.

dementia and the chapter has briefly reviewed four of the most common sub-types, their risk factors and protective factors. In the opening section of the chapter some clarity is also given to the meaning of Alzheimer's disease since the way Alzheimer's disease is conceptualized has changed significantly over time. How *dementia* differs from other conditions such as *MCI* and *age-related memory loss problems* has also been outlined.

The second part of the chapter advanced to a discussion of dementia policy in Ireland. In this section, new incidence and prevalence rates of dementia for Ireland were presented, information on the cost of care was provided and an overview was given on the political context underpinning the development of Irish health and social care policy in the field of dementia services. The strategic role the Atlantic Philanthropies has played in bringing fiscal and political attention to a health condition and disability previously under-prioritized in Ireland has been highlighted in the final part of the chapter. In this way this introductory chapter has set the context for the chapters to follow in this book.

CHAPTER 2

Models of dementia care

Introduction

This chapter explores the important topic of how different models for representing dementia can enhance insights and can help drive change in dementia policy practice and research. Models are tools or aids used to help us better understand what might otherwise appear as complex phenomena. Traditionally in Ireland the biomedical model that focused exclusively on a neuropathological explanation of dementia, dominated public discourse. The chapter argues that the biomedical model with its emphasis on pathology, disease, plaques, tangles and drug treatments is limiting and restrictive. Increasingly there is recognition that the clinical features of the diseases that cause dementia are also influenced by other variables including social factors. Likewise, there is increasing recognition that by reframing dementia in broader social, public health and rights-based terms, much can be done to improve the lives of all people living with and affected by the condition. So how can models be used to broaden the debate on Alzheimer's disease and dementia and what are the strengths and weaknesses of the well-known biomedical model?

The biomedical model

The biomedical model for framing dementia is the model with which most people are familiar. This model is said to gain its strength and appeal from classical science, from values such as objectivity and from the resources and expertise of the medical profession and pharmaceutical industries (Sabat, 2010). The biomedical model focuses largely on diseases that need to be fixed, treated, cured or at least rehabilitated and drug treatments are considered the main solution to multiple health problems.

In the context of dementia, those who subscribe to the biomedical model, consider the person predominantly from a diseased and atrophied brain perspective with little attention paid to that person's emotional social and cultural well-being (Vernooij-Dassen, 2019). Dementia is by and large regarded as a neurodegenerative brain disorder and a diagnosis based on history-taking, a neurological examination, blood screening, neuroimaging, electroencephalogram (EEG), cerebrospinal fluid (CSF) analysis and cognitive assessment is a prerequisite for medical treatments. A diagnosis is also necessary for accessing most health and social care service supports.

From a research perspective, the biomedical model reflects a positivist approach that places a strong emphasis on quantitative research methodology, randomized controlled trials and direct causal explanations: the personal narrative or subjective experience is not given that much consideration. For example, in drug trials, success is measured, not by eliciting the views of the individual and their experiences of drug use but instead by using validated scales to measure changes over time in domains such as memory, cognition, language, quality of life, executive functioning and so on (Diaz-Ponce, 2014). As noted by Sabat (2010, p. 93), 'the biomedical voice prizes and reflects the objective measurements of people's cognitive abilities as defined by the assets and limitations of standard testing'. The evolution of Irish health and social care services for people with dementia has been strongly influenced by the biomedical model where it has been noted that systems have traditionally been clinician-led and services medicalized and custodial (O'Shea et al., 2019).

While the biomedical model can help to explain the cause of memory, cognitive, functional and behavioural problems and through drug treatments offers hope, it has several limitations (Bond, 2001; Vogt et al., 2014). First, dementia defies biomedical thinking (Hughes, 2011) since a disconnect often exists between symptoms and brain pathology (Snowden, 2001; Vernooij-Dassen et al., 2019). As cited by Vernooij-Dassen and colleagues (2019), one study, some years ago, showed that almost 50% of elderly people with dementia had insufficient brain neuropathology to explain their symptoms (Balasubramanian et al., 2012) and another study (Corrada et al., 2012) has shown that high levels of pathology were present in about one third of older people who had no symptoms of dementia. Second, dementia is neither entirely preventable nor curable (Livingston et al., 2017). Third, with its primary focus on deficits, shrunken brains, neurocognitive testing and behavioural and psychological symptoms, the biomedical model assumes a linear relationship between pathology and disease. It fails to consider *the patient* as an active partner in the treatment process (Sabat, 2018).

Despite such limitations, the biomedical model has played a critical role in providing treatments that in a minority of cases may temporarily slow down cognitive decline and address dementia-related behavioural and psychological effects. Biomedical research has also led to an enhanced understanding of the ageing brain and to theories about aging and dementia (Vernooij-Dassen et al., 2019). A timely diagnosis is also a prerequisite to receiving interventions including drug treatments and psychological and social supports, which may improve the trajectory of symptoms and the individual's and family ability to cope.

The social model

A counter frame for understanding dementia is the social model: one that builds on the social model of disability (Oliver, 1983; Bond, 2001) and that carefully distinguishes between terms such as *impairment* and *disability*. While *impairment* refers to a condition of the mind or body, *disability* refers to how society can create inabilities by failing to effectively respond to a person's impairment. Proponents of the social model claim that solutions for the individual can be found, not in tackling or curing the impairment (a biological explanation), but rather by dismantling the artificial barriers society erects against people who have the impairment (a social explanation). So, for example, by adapting the built environment and making it more accessible through cueing and signage, the person diagnosed can be empowered to live more independently. Likewise, by adapting the psychosocial environment through challenging the at times discriminatory attitudes of others, a person living with dementia may be given increased agency and be enabled to live a more fulfilling and dignified life.

The social model does not diminish the importance of biomedical approaches but recognizes that dementia is also a disability (Bartlett, 2000; Kitwood, 1997a), solutions to which can be found in reducing some of the 'excess disabilities' (Sabat, 1994) society creates and the person experiences. The social model also emphasizes the way in which the individual and their family members interpret their experiences; the meaning their situation has for them and the efforts they make to participate as social citizens in society (Bond, 2001). This model has been heavily critiqued for many reasons, not least for its capacity to overlook the way in which impairments can significantly affect a person's quality of life (Degener, 2014). Although some people diagnosed with dementia are reluctant to acknowledge *having a disability* in addition to *having dementia* (Mental Health Foundation, 2015), the model is being used by advocacy groups such as Dementia Alliance International (DAI, 2016) and by dementia Working Groups across the world.

In Ireland the HSE's 'Understand Together' programme (see Chapter 1) provides a good exemple of the successful implementation of the social model of dementia. The campaign places a strong emphasis on public and professional education, on community awareness of dementia and on social engagement, connectivity, participation and social inclusion. There are other examples of the social model at play in the Irish dementia service landscape, several of which will be expanded on in Chapter 3 of this book. They include: (i) the earlier delivery of more personalized and flexible respite care services through the HSE and Genio's dementia programme (Cahill et al., 2014a), (ii) the development and delivery of a dementia advisory service by the ASI and (iii) the recent introduction and evaluation of post-diagnostic support services for community-dwelling people with dementia (Pierce et al., 2019). Examples like these provide evidence of a less deficit-based, less clinical and more person-centred model of dementia care gradually gaining traction in a country, where in the past, dementia services were task-focused and underpinned by a more conventional biomedical model.

The biopsychosocial model

Building on Tom Kitwood's pioneering work (1993a,b, 1997a,b) a more holistic approach to understanding dementia which brings together the strengths of both the biomedical model and social model has more recently been identified (see, e.g., Hughes, 2011, 2014; Sabat, 2011; Spector et al., 2016; Revolta et al., 2016 and Clare, 2017). Referred to as the biopsychosocial model, this approach points to the importance of considering the broad range of factors: biological, psychological, social, economic, cultural and environmental which are likely to influence the subjective experience of dementia.

The biopsychosocial model expands on the social model by placing a greater emphasis on the myriad of factors, social and non-social, likely to influence the individual's experience of an illness. It adopts a 'whole person' approach to dementia and recognizes the multiple domains – behavioural, functional, physical, psychological and emotional likely to be affected by dementia. In so doing it demonstrates that no single specialty has the expertise to respond to the multiple challenges that dementia poses. Rather the optimal approach, to enable the individual live well, is through involvement of multiple skilled personnel including, nurse practitioner, medical doctor, occupational therapist, social worker, psychologist, speech and language therapist, physiotherapist, dietician and so on.

This biopsychosocial model is well aligned with the newly emerging philosophy of reablement (Mishra and Barratt, 2016), an approach which challenges negative discourse (George, 2010). Rather than homing in on deficits and decline, this model builds on strengths and retained abilities and promotes autonomy, independence, choice and control. The biopsychosocial model is not necessarily clinician-led. It requires close collaboration between medical and nursing personnel, allied health care staff, the individual, care workers and family members. The approach is person-centred and strengths based. The biopsychosocial model when applied to the everyday life of a person whether at home, in acute care or in residential care also promotes acceptance, inclusion and awareness. It highlights what people can still achieve irrespective of the severity of dementia. It shifts the focus from frameworks that are task-focused and ignore subjectivity to those that are value driven and holistic.

The citizenship model

Another model for understanding dementia that is gradually gaining traction over the last decade is the citizenship model (Bartlett and O'Connor, 2007, 2010; Bartlett, 2014; Nedlund et al., 2019; Seetharaman and Chaudhury, 2020). The early description of citizenship dates back to the mid-eighteenth century and to the French Revolution when the idea was first linked to inequality, discrimination and to power relations in society (Bartlett and O'Connor, 2007). Since then 'citizenship' has been used in cognate disciplines especially in disability studies to make seemingly personal struggles political and public and to promote the status of discriminated groups enabling them to gain equity and agency. While in the context of dementia, the social and biopsychosocial models, focus on personhood and on the individual's perspective, the citizenship model focuses on society and on its socio-political structures that may promote or deny an individual's rights as a citizen. Analysing dementia using a citizenship lens broadens the debate and forces us to think about people with dementia as equal citizens who are entitled to the same from life as everyone else (Bartlett and O'Connor, 2010).

Bartlett and O'Connor (2010) have further expanded on the original citizenship model by proposing a *social citizenship* model of dementia. This refers to the 'relationship, practice or status, in which a person with dementia is entitled to experience freedom from discrimination and to have opportunities to grow and participate in life to the fullest extent possible' (p. 37). Central to this model are the concepts of: (i) *growth* – maximising resources to develop capacity, (ii) *social positions* – recognizing that people living with dementia have different positions in society and multiple identities, (iii) *purpose* – recognizing the importance of the individual becoming engaged and connected to people or things that provide purpose and meaning, (iv) *participation* – recognizing that people with dementia can take meaningful action and are agents of change, (v) *solidarity* – acknowledging the responsibility that people living with dementia have towards others who also have dementia and highlighting the importance of collective action as a society and (vi) *freedom from discrimination* – acknowledging the right to be treated fairly and not to be discriminated against or made feel different because of a diagnosis (Bartlett and O'Connor, 2010). The citizenship model especially the notion of *everyday citizenship* (see Nedlund et al., 2019) that shifts the emphasis away from care settings, diagnosis and post-diagnostic services to normal routines and events in a person's everyday life, broadens the agenda further. Although useful, application of the citizenship model becomes less salient with more advanced dementia (Bartlett and O'Connor, 2010).

The human rights model

Building on Degener's work (2014), where she proposes a human rights model of disability, in a similar vein, a human rights model of dementia can also help to reframe dementia in a more nuanced way. However, to date this model has not been well developed. Whilst the citizenship model of dementia hones in on first generational rights or civil and political rights such as the right to be treated equally before the law and the right to fully participate in all aspects of everyday life; people with dementia also need their social, economic and cultural rights (second generational rights) to be respected and upheld. Accordingly, the human rights model of dementia takes cognizance of both sets of rights and in this way is more comprehensive (Cahill, 2018a).

The human rights model of dementia also focuses on the dignity of the individual; it requires governments to treat all people as equal and never to discriminate. The model builds on the social model of dementia by moving beyond supporting anti-discriminatory policy, to supporting economic policies and social policies that ensure that the person can exercise choice and control over their everyday life and can enjoy a good quality of life despite having dementia. Whilst the social model has been critiqued for its neglect of pain and impairment (Degener, 2014) the human rights model acknowledges that impairments exist that can cause pain, distress, frustration, discomfort, stigma and so on. Cognitive impairment can cause a significant decline in how a person thinks, acts, feels and behaves. It can lead to frustration, anxiety and social isolation and can adversely affect that individual's quality of life.

Unlike the social model of disability that is critical of prevention policy, since a policy on the prevention of impairment may be regarded as a: 'policy of eliminating disabled persons' (Degener, 2014, p. 23), the human rights model considers that prevention policy is critically important. In the context of dementia, prevention of cognitive impairment (primary prevention), early detection and screening (secondary prevention) and the possible slowing down of dementia through lifestyle choices and risk reduction (tertiary prevention) (Wu et al., 2015) constitute important policy objectives in many countries' dementia strategies (Pot and Petrea, 2013; WHO, 2017). In the NDS, both the prevention of dementia along with health and social care service development remain key policy objectives.

Lastly, the human rights model also offers a road map for political and social change. The tools for change can be found in several human rights instruments including the UN Convention on the Rights of Persons with Disabilities (CRPD, 2006). This instrument has the potential to offer legal protection (Article 12), service entitlement (Article 19) and can change public understanding of dementia (Article 8). Reflecting the interconnectivity of human rights some of the Articles contained in the UN Convention, incorporate civil and political rights alongside social and economic rights. For a more detailed overview of this topic on dementia and human rights, see Cahill, 2018a.

A public health approach

Finally, a public health approach to framing dementia is also gaining momentum especially through the work of WHO (2012, 2016), the Alzheimer's Disease International (ADI, 2015) and the Organization for Economic Co-operation and Development (OECD, 2015) and according as more information becomes available about risk reduction and primary prevention (Winblad et al., 2016). The public health approach considers the broader set of factors, social, economic and environmental likely to influence health. Government action that involves structural interventions is required to address the challenge of dementia. This includes advocacy and consciousness raising, policy implementation, health and social care service response, capacity building, carer support and research (WHO, 2012).

Proponents of a public health approach argue that brain health and cognitive health in ageing are embedded in physical and mental health in earlier years so that from the point of view of public policy, every stage in the life course matters (Wu et al., 2016). The public health approach offers a paradigm of hope and optimism by helping to combat stigma and by severing the conventional association held between dementia and ageing and between mental health and dementia. This approach is strongly embedded in the WHO's global action plan on dementia (2017).

The public health approach acknowledges that many known diseases causing dementia, such as Alzheimer's disease and vascular disease, share the same characteristics of other chronic diseases. These include, a complex aetiology, multiple risk factors, long latency period, prolonged illness trajectory and result in functional impairment or disability (Travers et al., 2015). This means that the health promotion interventions applied to other diseases such as coronary heart disease, stroke, diabetes, cancer and chronic obstructive pulmonary disease may also be applicable to dementia. This also means that economies of effort can be gained through the promotion of health promotion policies (Travers et al., 2015) and it also means that public health policies targeting whole populations such as risk reduction and health promotion are important for dementia.

Whilst the NDS makes explicit reference to the importance of including dementia in all future health policies, dementia is not listed as a condition in the HSE's chronic disease management programme (<http://health.gov.ie/future-health/reforming-primary-care-2/managing-chronic-disease/>) nor is dementia a listed condition in the HSE's new chronic disease management programme for GPs. Likewise, dementia does not feature in any significant way in Ireland's healthy ageing programmes including in the Positive Ageing Strategy (DOH, 2013). Within the HSE, there are opportunities now for new partnerships to be developed between organizations that promote similar risk reduction messages for other chronic diseases. The recent setting up of a national working group on primary prevention and risk reduction for dementia, comprising staff from the NDO along with those from the HSE's *health and well-being programme* provides one useful example of these type of partnerships.

Conclusions

This chapter has described a range of models, biomedical, social, biopsychosocial, citizenship and human rights that can be used to broaden our understanding of dementia. Each model each has its strengths and weaknesses, and none is without limitation. The biomedical model may one day help to find a cure or fully effective treatment for dementia, but it is restrictive, as it tells only one part of the overall story. The social model helps us better understand the artificial barriers society can erect that make life harder for a person living with dementia, but it fails to consider the multiple impairments a person with dementia may experience and how impairments can adversely affect the individual's life.

The citizenship model places an emphasis on civil and political rights such as the right to legal capacity or the right to vote in an election but overlooks economic, social and cultural rights. The human rights model although currently under-developed, provides a more nuanced understanding of dementia but to be fully implemented, this approach will require significant resources. The biopsychosocial model, laudable for its recognition of the multiple domains likely to be affected by dementia and the multiple stakeholders likely to be involved in dementia care, may not be that helpful in the real world, where there will always be jockeying for position amongst clinicians and other health service professionals for ownership and expertise in dementia care. The magnitude of dementia is such that we need to draw on the strengths and insights provided by each of these models and work collaboratively to achieve more holistic and optimal results.

As discussed in this chapter, how dementia is understood in Ireland has changed significantly over a relatively short period in time. Evidence is now emerging of a gradual dismantling of the biomedical model, that viewed dementia predominantly as a cognitive brain disorder and the emergence of a person-centred community-based model with a focus on personhood and citizenship. Part of this transformation has been driven by the Atlantic Philanthropies' investment programme in dementia in Ireland. Another part has been influenced by the government's implementation of the NDS (DOH, 2014). The dismantling of a strongly embedded biomedical model of dementia has significant implications for service development and demands a whole person multidisciplinary response to dementia. It acknowledges the need to provide not only medical interventions but also a broad range of social care services including rehabilitation and other post-diagnostic supports. Several of these service supports will now be reviewed in the chapter to follow.

CHAPTER 3

Diagnostic and post-diagnostic services

Introduction

This chapter explores the topic of the diagnosis and disclosure of dementia and why obtaining a diagnosis is critically important. It also addresses the question of who within the medical profession in Ireland has responsibility for the diagnosis and disclosure of dementia and what constitutes best practice in this area. Living well with dementia requires psychological and emotional adjustment, often facilitated by high quality services, so what type of post-diagnostic supports are available to people in Ireland recently diagnosed? What is the evidence base for these services and how does Ireland compare with other European countries in relation to the provision of post-diagnostic supports? Is there an ideal model of post-diagnostic service support that might best target the complex needs of people diagnosed? These along with other important questions will be addressed in this chapter – but first to a cautionary note about the use of language in discussions about dementia diagnosis.

Early versus timely diagnosis.

Nowadays policy makers and medical doctors talk about the importance of a *timely diagnosis* rather than an *early diagnosis* of dementia. While the terms *timely* and *early* are often used interchangeably, for the purpose of this chapter, I use these terms to refer to a diagnosis that ideally occurs at the right time and sufficiently early to enable the individual and family members participate in legal, financial and future care planning. This is how I interpret these terms, but it is important to note that others have a different interpretation. For example, for some, an *early diagnosis* is understood to mean a diagnosis made as early as possible in a chronological sense (Dhedi et al., 2014; AE, 2016).

De Lepeleire et al. (2008) were probably one of the first to use the word *timely* to mean: that time when the individual or caregiver and doctor recognize that dementia may be developing. Their preference for the word *timely* in the context of a diagnosis, suggests that the focus should be on making a speedy response to the first reported signs of changed behaviour and functioning rather than on population screening and making the earliest possible diagnosis.

Others define *timely* to mean that time when the benefits of diagnosis outweigh risks (Nuffield Council on Bioethics, 2009) or the optimum time for the individual and family members to use information about a diagnosis to plan for the future (Brooker et al., 2014). The NDS (DOH, 2014) uses the word *timely* to mean a diagnosis that is: 'made and communicated at a time and in a way that best matches the physical, emotional, medical and other needs of the patient, their families and carers' (p. 20).

But before progressing to a discussion of who within the medical profession has responsibility for a timely diagnosis, it is important to comment about the time leading up to a diagnosis since a person may have symptoms of dementia or MCI for several years before a diagnosis is ever made.

Time prior to diagnosis

The pre-diagnostic phase of dementia can generate fear and uncertainty for the individual coping with the symptoms, (Steeman et al., 2006; Górska et al., 2018) and for family members (Rogers et al., 2017). Most of us have had the annoying experience of losing or mislaying important items like mobile phones, wallets, credit cards, keys and so on. But imagine if mislaying valuable items became a regular feature of everyday life to the extent that you were prevented from getting on with your life.

Imagine also if you started getting lost in familiar places or were forgetting the names of very familiar people or you were repeatedly letting your friends down, forgetting to turn up to important social events. Think about how embarrassed, frustrated and distressed you might feel! And although dementia impairs memory, behaviour and cognitive function, the amygdala or that part of the brain responsible for emotion remains intact. So, people with dementia are likely to still experience embarrassment, shame, alarm, frustration annoyance and so on.

Alzheimer's disease is also insidious (Shi et al., 2000): its signs and symptoms may fluctuate and a person may have both good days and bad. So, just as a close family member starts to believe they were imagining the symptoms noticed and all is well again, a further, more obvious decline in that person's abilities arises. Eventually when it becomes apparent that compared with in the past, a very significant deterioration in that person's memory, cognition, behaviour and social functioning has occurred, a decision must be made about obtaining medical advice.

Some families rush into making this decision for their relative in an effort to protect them. However, it should be remembered that the decision to obtain a diagnosis needs to be made by the person experiencing the symptoms or at the very least in conjunction with that person. If the person is resistant, they may be frightened and hesitant to confront the reality of an irreversible and often stigmatizing condition that cannot be effectively treated. They may need time and encouragement to confront this reality. Reminding the person of some of the potential benefits a timely diagnosis may yield may also be very helpful.

Benefits of a timely diagnosis

A burgeoning body of literature now exists demonstrating the multiple benefits an early/timely diagnosis is likely to confer[1] (see, e.g., ADI, 2011). Diagnosis has been referred to as the gateway to care (Knapp et al.,

---

[1] It needs to be remembered that there are risks associated with obtaining a diagnosis. These risks pertain to the doctor, the individual and family members. Risks for the medical doctor include their being incorrect or making a false positive diagnosis, for the family caregiver, their having to adopt a primary caregiving role prematurely and for the individual, stigma, loss of status, income, independence and dignity along with fear of being relegated to the status of a non-person in a society that places undue emphasis on sharp minds and cognitive capabilities (Hughes, 2014).

2007) and the identification of the dementia sub-type as the gateway to drug treatment (Iliffe et al., 2009). A diagnosis enables planning for the future, referral to relevant support services, the prescription of medication and may help to relieve the psychological distress often experienced by the individual and by caregivers (Foley et al., 2019). For the individual a diagnosis can signal an important transition from uncertainty and ambiguity to a new phase where the person can be supported to adapt to changes (Woods et al., 2003). The diagnosis can promote dignity and well-being by providing a plausible explanation behind what is causing the cognitive impairment or changed behaviour (Cahill and Shapiro, 1997). A diagnosis can also maximize autonomy (ADI, 2011) by allowing the person to participate in decision-making at a time when their capacity is still intact.

Drug treatments like cholinesterase inhibitors (see Chapter 1) and non-drug treatments like cognitive rehabilitation and cognitive stimulation therapy (see later part of this chapter) are said to have maximum effect during the early stages of dementia (Milne, 2010; Brooker et al., 2014). Legal and financial planning such as in Ireland, appointing an assistant decision-maker (ADM) or co-decision-maker (CDM) or making an advanced health care directive (statement made about decision-making on treatments and health care) or taking out an enduring powers of attorney (EPA) (nominating a trusted person to act on one's behalf in relation to complex decision-making, when one's decision-making ability is compromised) can only be drawn up when the person still has insight and capacity (see Chapter 6). Some individuals will want to know their diagnosis because giving a name to a health problem causing disabling symptoms provides a framework for understanding. Accordingly given the importance of making a diagnosis, who has responsibility within the medical profession to diagnose?

Diagnosis

Different countries use different approaches to diagnose dementia. However, in most countries including Ireland, the GP is usually the first port of call for a person worried about their memory and cognitive symptoms (Foley et al., 2019; Heintz et al., 2020). GPs vary in motivation, ability, confidence and resources to diagnose dementia and for most GPs making the diagnosis is not straightforward (Buntinex et al., 2011) given that no definitive test is available (Workman et al., 2010). The Alcove study that surveyed experts across twenty-four EU countries concluded that GPs, neurologists, geriatricians and psychiatrists were the main professional groups involved in diagnosis but noted that specialist in-put was less common (Brooker et al., 2014).

Like in other countries, Irish government policy asserts that GPs play a pivotal role in the diagnosis and support of people with dementia. The NDS states: 'the general practitioner (GP) is usually the first contact when concerns about thinking or memory arise. The GP role involves identifying those symptoms indicative of dementia, excluding any other possible diagnoses and referring on to specialist services. GPs will also have an ongoing role supporting their patients and their families throughout their illness' (DOH, 2014, p. 20). Yet historically GPs in Ireland have not been trained to diagnose nor to disclose dementia (Cahill et al., 2006) despite calls for their upskilling in this area for many years (O'Shea and O'Reilly, 1999; Pierce, 2019).

Probably in response to such calls and as part of the implementation of the NDS, in 2015, the HSE and the Atlantic Philanthropies provided researchers based in University College Cork, with funding to the value of €1.2 million, for the Primary Care Education Pathways and Research in Dementia (PREPARED) project. This project was undertaken over a three-year period[2]. It was based on a range of inter-related professional activities that concerned four key areas namely: (i) clinical guidelines on dementia for general practice (Foley et al., 2019), (ii) the design and delivery of dementia education and training for GPs and primary care teams, (iii) the use of information technology to support GP decision-making (<www.dementiapathays.ie>) and (iv) the development of local dementia care

---

2   The PREPARED project is a GP-led project based in the Department of General Practice at University College Cork. It is led by Dr Tony Foley, an experienced and practising GP with a specialist interest in dementia, and a lecturer in general practice at University College Cork. It is supported by a team of GPs, researchers and a project manager working in the Department of General Practice at University College Cork.

pathways (Pierce, 2019). It built on an earlier specialist programme – the Kinsale Community Response to Dementia (K-CORD[3]) that was also funded through the Atlantic Philanthropies and Genio. The outputs from PREPARED have been extensive. Nationally over 500 GPs have attended small group peer-facilitated dementia workshops. One of the project's key findings is that to be effective, educational interventions need to be peer-facilitated with case-based discussions taking place in small interactive workshops (Foley, 2017).

Since the completion of PREPARED and with a desire to plan more equitable diagnostic services, a number of related projects committed to developing dementia care pathways have been implemented through the NDO. One of these, *the dementia diagnostic pathway project*, has several components, one of which was a literature review of the evidence base for diagnostic services (Revez et al., 2018). A conclusion reached based on this review was that for Ireland, flexibility is needed regarding dementia diagnostic service systems and that no *one size fits all* approach should be adopted. Apart from the recommendation that atypical and difficult to diagnose individuals should be assessed at specialist services, this review is non-prescriptive about which service sectors should have responsibility for which patient categories. It states that the local context needs consideration and a range of different assessment and diagnostic models are important. Potential settings of diagnostic services identified include: (i) regional memory clinics, (ii) local memory clinics, (iii) primary care and (iv) community mental health services.

Disclosure

An important part of the diagnostic process is the disclosure of the diagnosis to the individual since in the absence of disclosure, most aspects of post-diagnostic support including medication and referral to health

3   K-CORD the Kinsale community response to dementia was a primary care based project committed to heightening awareness of dementia and educating primary care staff about dementia. Through K-CORD diagnostic guidelines for GPs were developed along with an online dementia eLearning course.

and social care services are obstructed (Revez et al., 2018). Historically it was thought that disclosure to the individual might lead to high rates of depression, anxiety and suicidal ideation but these beliefs have more recently been overturned (Mormont et al., 2014). Today with some few exceptions, the disclosure by a medical doctor of a diagnosis to the 'patient' is considered good practice (Winblad et al., 2016). Best practice also suggests that information about the diagnosis should be communicated to the person in a gradual, progressive and supportive way and that disclosure should ideally be a therapeutic event rather than a horrific experience (Prince, 2015). A recent systematic review and meta-analysis that included findings from twenty-three studies demonstrated that 85% of people with symptoms of cognitive impairment or dementia (or those who were attending a memory clinic), favoured disclosure of their diagnosis (van den Dungen et al., 2014).

There has been a tendency in Ireland for GPs not to disclose the diagnosis of dementia to their patients (Cahill et al., 2006) or to use euphemisms when conveying the news (Begley, 2009). This avoidance has probably been based on the principle of beneficence or non-maleficence. However, the practice is at odds with those of several other European countries where disclosure to the person has been the norm for some time (Braekhus and Engedal, 2002). The practice of non-disclosure to the person has failed to consider the individual's personhood dignity and autonomy (see Chapter 6). Recent Irish research conducted with a sample of older hospital patients (all cognitively intact) found that the majority (86%) claimed they would like to know their diagnosis if they developed dementia (Robinson et al., 2014). We do not know how well or how inadequately disclosure is currently being managed by GPs or other clinicians in Ireland. However, based on a recent Irish study of young-onset dementia (Fox et al, 2020) a major disconnect was found between how well clinicians believed they communicated the news of dementia to their 'patient' and family members versus how unsatisfactory that communication was from the 'patient' and family members' perspective.

At diagnosis and disclosure, peoples' information needs are extensive (Begley, 2009; Diaz-Ponce, 2014; DOH, 2014). They need information about the dementia and its sub-type, disease progression and its prognosis, the effectiveness of drug treatments and side effects and the impact of other interventions such as assistive technologies, home adaptations, local social support services and advocacy services (Begley, 2009; AE, 2014). Information and advice are also often required about practical issues such as driving, money-management and legal matters. If the person diagnosed is still employed, information may also be required about how cognitive impairments are likely to impact on work performance. Also, if working hours need to be cut or an early retirement secured because of dementia, information will be required on income supports and pension/superannuation entitlements. If the person has a young-onset dementia, information may also be required on genetic testing and counselling. Accordingly, with such extensive information and support needs the person and their family will need a broad range of post-diagnostic services.

Post-diagnostic services

So, what exactly are post-diagnostic supports? Stated simply they refer to a range of service supports designed to enable people to live well in the community following a diagnosis. Although important for the individual and family member, post-diagnostic supports also have appeal for policy makers since their goal is to help delay admission to long-term residential care (SCIE, 2014). To be effective, post-diagnostic services need to be informative and useful. They must signpost people to the correct community-based services (Mayrhofer et al., 2018). Interestingly, it is not unusual for people living with dementia and their family members to express dissatisfaction with post-diagnostic services. One study has shown that what was problematic for several was: lack of communication, poor guidance, inadequate information and a general lack of support for living life well with dementia (Brodaty, 2019).

While traditionally in Ireland, services such as day care and residential respite care focused on family caregivers' needs and if available were offered during the more moderate to advanced stages of dementia, there is now increasing recognition of the diverse and complex needs the person will have immediately following a diagnosis. Within the international literature, there is also increasing support for the view that following a diagnosis, people want new and different services. They want services that are empowering, that support the individual in decision-making and help them manage the emotional and psychological impact of the diagnosis (Clarke et al., 2013). People also need services that can help them regain a sense of normality (von Kutzleben et al., 2012; Diaz-Ponce, 2014) and that offer peer support.

Globally much has also been written about post-diagnostic support services (OECD, 2015; WHO, 2012, 2017). The topic has also been carefully addressed in many countries' dementia policy plans. For example, one work stream of the English Strategy was the development of more individualized supports including dementia advisors and peer supports (Clarke et al., 2013). Scotland's second National Dementia Strategy focused specifically on improving post-diagnostic support for people living with dementia (SNDS, 2013) and since 2013, all Scottish people are guaranteed a minimum of twelve months dementia services post diagnosis. The Irish Strategy is thin on its commitment and clarity to post-diagnostic supports but states: '[a] person with dementia and their carer(s) need a clearly signposted pathway that directs them to the right care and support, in the right place and at the right time' (DOH, 2014, p. 25).

Models of post-diagnostic services

There is no gold standard or optimal model of post-diagnostic service support for people with dementia (Watts et al., 2013). This is not surprising given the heterogeneity and complexities of dementia, the fact that a diagnosis may occur at any stage in the course of the condition and that many older people will have co-morbidities possibly causing them more distress than dementia. However, information about dementia, treatments, support in signposting the individual to relevant services, peer support, planning for future care and future decision-making are considered mainstays of such services (AS, 2011). Clare (2002) argues that post-diagnosis support should also include activities that provide social contact to reduce social isolation and promote self-esteem. Others (Keady et al., 2007; Clarke et al., 2013) suggest the supports may help people come to terms with their diagnosis.

For some time now, deficits in post-diagnostic service supports for people living with dementia have been highlighted in small-scale Irish research studies (Begley, 2009; Bobersky, 2013; Diaz-Ponce, 2014), commissioned reports (O'Shea et al., 1999; Cahill et al., 2012) and more recently in submissions to the Slaintecare report (Oireachtas Committee on the Future of Health Care, 2017). This is not surprising given that historically Irish people have tended not to be told their diagnosis and service supports have traditionally focused on the needs of the primary caregiver and not on the everyday challenges facing the individual experiencing the symptoms (Cahill et al., 2014a).

To address these service deficits and as part of the advancement of the NDS, *a post-diagnostic grant scheme* was announced by the NDO in 2017. Drawing on dormant accounts, the scheme was designed to develop and implement a range of new supports across the country and increase staff capacity in their delivery. This new programme of support was preceded by a literature review that examined the research evidence. In synthesizing the literature, it was concluded that a broad range of post-diagnostic dementia supports are available that have potential to improve quality of life. These include: information and advice, psycho-educational supports, peer-support activities, cognitive rehabilitation (CR), cognitive stimulation therapy (CST), reminiscence and so on (O'Shea et al., 2018). Some post-diagnostic supports were shown to have a stronger evidence base than others.

Building on this literature review and a needs-analysis, three post-diagnostic service supports namely: (i) cognitive rehabilitation (CR) (ii) cognitive stimulation therapy (CST) and (iii) psychosocial educational interventions (PEI) were identified for trial in Ireland. Following open competition, grants were awarded to eighteen applicants, many of whom were HSE staff, to deliver at least one intervention over an eighteen-month period. The new post-diagnostic service supports were made available to a total of 232 people and 140 family caregivers in nine community health organizations[4]. An in-depth evaluation of this new post-diagnostic grant scheme was undertaken in the early stages of its implementation (Pierce et al., 2019).

The final part of this chapter will now review the evidence base for the three post-diagnostic service interventions selected, how and to whom these services were delivered and key findings emerging from the evaluation. This part of the chapter will also review the dementia advisory service introduced by the ASI over recent years since this new service also provides post-diagnostic supports.

Cognitive rehabilitation

Cognitive rehabilitation (CR) is an individualized problem-solving therapy that aims to reduce or manage functional disability by addressing personal goals selected by the individual diagnosed with dementia (Clare et al., 2019). The therapist usually starts with issues important to the person (the goal) such as handling money, remembering names, finding lost items and so on and then identifies that person's capacity and level of functioning. Following assessment to identify what is needed to attain this goal, evidence-based rehabilitation methods are used to design a plan. Although the evidence base for CR remains weak, its use is growing. Trials show that it has the potential to form a valuable component of post-diagnostic services, especially for people with early-stage dementia (Clare et al., 2013; Kelly and O'Sullivan 2015; Kim, 2015; Amieva et al., 2016). The largest recently completed trial (Clare et al., 2019) found that individual goal-oriented CR enabled community-dwelling people to function better and remain more independent in relation to their identified goals (Pierce et al., 2019). Compared with other countries, CR services are hugely under-developed in Ireland.

---

4   The scheme was not intended to target a large number of people diagnosed with dementia but rather its goal was to test the implementation of the programme with a view towards scaling it up at a later stage.

Commencing in late 2018, six CR programmes were delivered to eighty people living with dementia in different parts of the country through the NDO's post-diagnostic grant scheme. In advance of these programmes, masterclasses in CR were offered to interested and eligible service providers most of whom were occupational therapists. The CR provided focused mainly on memory rehabilitation and was delivered in group format. Despite the fact that the evidence base for CR is weak, participants rated it very positively (Pierce et al., 2019), a finding which may reflect the level of need experienced. Participants talked about the value of CR: they appreciated the information, practical advice and reassurance given. Solutions identified also helped many people to better manage their everyday life including activities of daily living. Peer support was an important component of CR and most participants said the intervention inspired confidence. Based on this evaluation a decision has been made to support the continuation of several of these CR programmes during 2020 (Emer Begley, personal communication, February 2020).

Cognitive stimulation therapy

Cognitive stimulation therapy (CST) has its roots in reality orientation (Woods et al., 2012). It is a group-based intervention consisting of structured sessions often held over prolonged periods (Kelly et al., 2017). The therapy targets cognitive or social functioning, has a social element and includes activities that stimulate thinking concentration and memory (O'Shea et al., 2018). CST has been shown to be more cost-effective than usual care (Knapp et al., 2006) and as effective as anti-dementia drugs (ADI, 2011). CST has been endorsed by the National Institute for Clinical Excellence in their guidelines for dementia and cognitive symptoms (NICE/SCIE, 2006; NICE, 2018). In the UK the intervention is considered a standard post-diagnostic support and is available free through the NHS. Also in the UK, access to CST is a mandatory requirement for all memory clinic accreditation (Martin Orrell, personal communication, January 2020). However, in Ireland, memory clinic accreditation is not mandatory and at the

Diagnostic and post-diagnostic services 43

time of writing, CST is not available at or accessible to most memory clinics. CST is available in about half of all EU countries, although variations exist in relation to criteria used for accessing the therapy free of charge (AE, 2014). The international evidence base for CST is significantly more robust than that for CR.

Commencing in late 2018, seven new CST programmes were delivered to eighty-nine Irish people diagnosed with dementia. Programmes were group-based and all but one was developed in line with the UK-based manual titled: 'Making a Difference CST Programme' (Aguirre et al., 2012). Programme evaluation revealed that CST was considered of great value to participants living with dementia and their family caregivers. Staff reported that for successful programme delivery, specialist training was needed as was the availability of two facilitators. This evaluation showed that CST can also be delivered in hospital settings and has the potential to benefit those with more advanced dementia. A conclusion reached was that CST was worth scaling up in Ireland. Several of these CST programmes will continue to be funded and available in 2020 (Emer Begley, personal communication, February 2020).

Psychosocial educational interventions

The third type of post-diagnostic support made available through the NDO was a psychosocial educational intervention (PEI). These interventions combine skills-training, peer support, psychological therapies and counselling and are different from support groups since they have an educational and therapeutic component (O'Shea et al., 2018). The educational component focuses on imparting information and knowledge about different aspects of dementia. The therapeutic component focuses on supporting the person manage illness-related circumstances. For the family caregiver, other known benefits of PEI include a reduction in caregiver burden, enhanced emotional well-being and reduced depression/anxiety (Pierce et al., 2019). PEI is said to be most beneficial when the family caregiver is separated from the person living with dementia during the intervention (Milne et al., 2014).

As part of the NDO's post-diagnostic support grant scheme, seven PEI's were delivered to sixty-three community-dwelling people living with dementia and seventy-six family caregivers during 2019. Programmes were designed to provide practical information and upskill people on topics including social connectedness, peer support, decision-making and future care planning. The programmes, four of which were group-based and the remainder individual, were run once weekly over a four to six-week period. They were delivered by staff from a wide range of professional backgrounds. The evaluation found great variability across the country: the most successful programme was an intervention that took place over a four-week period and involved a joint weekly meeting between a health service professional, the person diagnosed with dementia and their family caregiver (Pierce et al., 2019). This programme of post-diagnostic interventions will continue to be funded and offered in parts of the country during 2020.

Dementia advisors

Navigating the dementia care system is complex (Clarke et al., 2013) and information and support services are needed at the right time, in the right place and in the right format. Some of the challenges that confront the individual and family members include fragmented care; poorly integrated health and social care systems and the involvement of multiple agencies and many different providers (AE, 2014). This can often result in assessment duplication and confusion. To support people to navigate the health and social care system, dementia advisors also referred to as key workers, link workers, or case managers have been available in some countries as for example, in Scotland, England, France, the Netherlands and Australia. In several of these countries, the role of dementia advisor has evolved in different ways. For example, in France, the dementia advisor is more of a case manager, while in Australia, that person is usually a health service professional who has a significant training and educational remit (de Siún, 2013). In Ireland, a distinction is made between the role of case manager and dementia advisor. The case manager is allegedly employed within the health and social care system and has responsibility for case management while the dementia advisor is employed by the ASI and has exclusive responsibility for referral and signposting to support services.

During 2014, the ASI piloted a new dementia advisory service in Dublin and Cork. The main aim of this service was to signpost families to relevant service supports and to work with individuals and families to provide timely information and support (ASI, 2019). For the individual, choice, control, empowerment and peer support were considered fundamental components of the service. Over time this ASI service has extended to cover the counties of Galway, Tipperary, Cork, Kerry, Clare and Limerick and it is now co-funded by the HSE. Findings from an evaluation of this service have shown that while individuals, family members and service providers were satisfied with this service, there was a need for greater clarity about the scope of the service and the precise role of dementia advisor (Coffey et al., 2018). There was also a need for better integration of the dementia advisor with pre-existing services and greater public awareness and coverage of the service. More recently the out-going government has agreed to support the expansion of this service by funding the appointment of ten additional dementia advisors.

Conclusions

Written against the backdrop of the NDS, this chapter has explored the topic of dementia diagnosis and disclosure and has addressed the important question of who within the medical profession in Ireland has responsibility for this. Like other countries around the world, the pivotal role Irish GPs play in diagnosing and disclosing dementia has been highlighted. In keeping with the theme of empowering the individual and always keeping that person at the centre stage, it is argued that the person experiencing the symptoms of dementia should always be involved in decision-making about obtaining a diagnosis. Some of the benefits an early diagnosis confers on the person have been highlighted.

The second part of the chapter advances to a discussion of the new programme of post-diagnostic service supports made available by the NDO to some people in Ireland. In this part of the chapter, a detailed account is given of the three service interventions namely CR, CST and PEI, funded through dormant accounts. This is an important new programme that has potential to be extended and embedded in the system. Its value lies not only in how it helps to support the individual and their family members but also in how the programme helps increase staff capacity in an area that has until recently been hugely overlooked. Although efforts to develop post-diagnostic services are now well underway, this new programme has relied on dormant accounts and at the moment it caters for only a small proportion of all those likely to be affected by dementia. This chapter has provided a useful backdrop for the one to follow that will now focus on the diagnostic and post-diagnostic experiences of one Irish person diagnosed with *young-onset dementia*.

CHAPTER 4

The journey to diagnosis and living with dementia: Still me

I have been asked to contribute to this book by telling my own personal story. The story starts some years back and I will tell it now as how I remember it.

In my early 40s I went through a spell of bad health. I was not working as I wanted to be at home with the guys (my two sons) until they started school. I mentioned to my GP that my recent memory was not as sharp as it had been. He explained that the brain is a muscle and it needs to be worked and challenged or it gets 'flabby'. So, I started doing puzzles: I also did random night classes and learned cross stitch.

Life went on and got busy and we fostered children. The guys got more involved in various sports and hobbies. I wanted a career change and started studying. My Mom had a very rough year before she died of lung cancer and during that time, I often dropped the guys to school, drove to Dublin (I am originally from Dublin) spent a few hours with her and then drove back to Cashel in time to collect them. Sadly, my marriage ended after several years of dealing with alcoholism. During that time one of my son's was dealing with some psychological issues.

My Dad was diagnosed with Vascular dementia and as time went on his visits to the house (he often spent weeks with us) were becoming difficult and sometimes distressing. It was hard to understand some of his behaviours and it could be disturbing when he became agitated. I did not know how best to support him or understand what was going on. It came to a stage where we had to question if for Dad, being away from his home was in his best interest, so I decided to go find that information.

At the time, the ASI ran a six-week course, one evening a week in Clonmel. Little did I know how far-reaching the effects of this would be! As I was doing the course, not only did I find that I myself had some of the symptoms being described, but I also had many strategies in place for things most people my age had no difficulty with. For example, I had a diary for keeping appointments and developed various routines to keep the house running smoothly. I had lists upon lists and pen and paper in every room. If I did not have a word to describe an object, I mimed an action and the guys responded. I spoke to one of the facilitators at the ASI and she had not noticed anything out of the ordinary in my behaviour, but she said if I was concerned to contact my GP and get myself checked out.

Prior to all of this, I had seen a documentary on TV about dementia. I found it so disturbing that I told my husband: 'if I was ever diagnosed with Alzheimer's, shoot me before I leave the surgery'. I had a very negative, poorly informed understanding of the disease. At that stage one of my sons was going through some tough stuff and I did not think I could deal with a diagnosis on top of everything else, so I tried to bury my head in the sand.

After many months the old Kathy kicked in and I started to question maybe there were breakthroughs in a cure or medications to slow down the progression. I spoke to my GP who knows me well and he laughed and said not you! He did the mini mental test examination (a test to detect memory and cognitive problems) that I failed miserably. So that was when I started my official journey to a diagnosis, a bumpy road to say the least!

I was referred to the local memory clinic. At the same time a new diabetic doctor (I also have diabetes) came to the local hospital. When I mentioned some of what was going on, that doctor decided to do a barrage of tests, including a scan. I then had my first assessment in the memory clinic in September 2013 which was inconclusive. I was referred to a neuropsychologist for a more in-depth assessment. I naively believed because of what I had read about plaques and tangles that if the brain scan was clear then it was not Alzheimer's disease: I was also told that whatever was causing my problems was not Alzheimer's disease. I had the second assessment in November 2013. I also have osteoporosis, so I have scans every few years.

My GP had requested a bone densitometry scan (DXA) and when I received an appointment for the X-ray department, I just assumed it was for the DXA. The writing on the form was illegible, but I knew I was not due for any other type of X-ray. That day when I went for the X-ray department I was asked to strip to my underwear. Now this was unusual for a DXA scan and so I queried it. The lady read my name, address, date of birth and my hospital number and all were correct. At that stage I asked what the X-ray was for and she told me that it was for my spine and chest. So I told her she had the wrong person. She then asked had I recently had a brain scan? I replied yes but why would they want to X-ray my spine and chest? The response and to this day it makes my blood run cold was: she told me they were checking that the cancer in my brain had not metastasized to my spine or lungs!

I then asked her to check with someone more senior to her about this. I sat scared to death. I was then told that yes, the head of the X-ray department wanted the X-rays done. So I agreed.

Afterwards I phoned my GP to check what was going on. I did not hear back until the next day. Needless to say I did not sleep a wink that night. Apparently, I had fluid on my brain something many people have and do not know they have it but at least I did not have the big C. That was in November 2013 and to say that I really enjoyed Christmas that year is an understatement. I did not have cancer or Alzheimer's disease; anything else seemed manageable! I wondered if the medication I was taking for my cholesterol could be causing the problem.

On the 23rd January 2014 I attended the local memory clinic for results. It was a small room with four or five people and I was told that I had mild cognitive impairment: something I had never heard of before. But the statement had 'mild' in there so that did not sound so bad after all. I then asked all the questions I thought were appropriate and left.

I came away thinking that was not so bad and planned on researching mild cognitive impairment. I was taking my son to Kilkenny for a meeting on the same day and was focusing on that. As I crossed the car park, I met the nurse a lovely lady, who had done the first assessment. She apologized to me for not being with me at my appointment and knew I did not have any support. I told her not to worry that I was fine and it was a good outcome. She apologized again saying that she had been called away in an emergency. At that moment I realized, either I had not heard something or something had not been said. So, I asked her straight out: 'do I have Alzheimer's disease'? The answer was yes.

I was shocked but knew I had to be ok as I was due to collect Andrew to take him to Kilkenny. My son has the ability to read your soul. She kindly offered to meet me for coffee the following week and I rushed off. I was confused, I thought that maybe she was wrong but I would deal with it later.

On the way to Kilkenny I got a call from the hospital asking if I would take medication. I agreed. Hours later I googled the medication I had been prescribed and to my horror it was for Alzheimer's disease. Then I knew I had it. It was like being slammed into a wall and there was no going back.

I was devastated, shaken, sad, angry, lost, I felt hopeless, afraid, alone, scared, so upset that I was bringing this into my sons' lives, who were both still so young. I felt like I was alternating between walking around in a dense fog, to hanging off a cliff by my fingernails. Yet in among all the negative feelings and emotions was relief – yes relief, strange as it sounds! Now there was a reason why I was unable to do some of the things, others like friends of my age, had no difficulty with. I knew I was not actually going bonkers!

At first, I chose not to tell my sons until I could make some sense out of things: but for how long what next and so on? When I look back there were many wet pillows, sleepless nights, many broken conversations where we would be chatting about the future and it would hit me like a ton of bricks: would I be around, would I recognize my sons, would I be locked inside my own head?

As a parent, it is very important to me to try to be a good role model. Many people have crap come into their lives. Some bad and tough things happen to all of us: this gave me time to come to terms with what was eventually going to control every aspect of my life. I needed to be as okay as possible with this before I told the guys as things I thought would never be the same again once I told them.

At the time, Andrew, my eldest son, was repeating his leaving certificate and Matt the younger boy has an anxiety disorder. I was not going to tell one without the other and certainly was not going to tell them prior to Andrew's exams. That time gave me space to explore Mr A, (Alzheimer's disease) gather information and focus on what I could do, to be as well as possible for as long as possible.

I was referred to a psychiatrist, who asked me if I was depressed and if so said it was ok to be depressed and there was no shame in taking medications for depression. The psychiatrist did not seem to believe me when I said I did not think I was, that I was ok with taking medications if I needed to and asked me to ask my GP did he think I was depressed. His response was a resounding no. I was then hearing things like I might not know my own children in three years' time and that I was probably further along than I thought, yaddi, yaddi yah! I realized that I was allowing some very negative thoughts and information take root. I was sitting in a pity parlour feeling very sorry for myself and that I was counting the days, weeks, occasions and in fact, just waiting for Mr A, the intruder, to take over. In short I had given up!

Again, the old Kathy kicked in. My faith has seen me through many tough times and I knew God would not abandon me. When I could not pray, I just sat in front of the tabernacle and slowly started to regain my peace. To this day the church is my 'go to' place when I am overwhelmed. I started to ask: what could I do about this and what could I learn and did I need to change my behaviour and attitude and what was God asking of me? So, I put 'post it' notes up all around the house saying INSTEAD OF COUNTING THE DAYS, MAKE EACH DAY COUNT. Something I have tried to do since as none of us are guaranteed tomorrow.

Looking back now, I realize that a huge part of this journey is about grieving. This grieving is ongoing from the very moment of diagnosis. I have learned that grieving is not only about death but also about loss, the loss of anything that is important to you. For those of us diagnosed with dementia, that grief and loss is a constant companion and not only for us but for our loved ones. Yet little is said about it.

My goal was always to go to college once the guys had finished school, to create some financial stability. I wanted to work in the area I was volunteering in but could not get paid for as I did not have a degree. So my goal was to see and do things I had long dreamed about. The loss of dreams, goals, abilities, joys, skills, sensory changes, fear of simple things you took for granted yesterday, last week, are all some form of loss, big and small. Sadly, I do not think there is enough counselling or grief work being done in this area, most especially for couples.

As time went on, I wondered did I really need to tell the guys yet. I queried this with my GP who felt that due to other health issues, the guys needed to hear it from me. Also, I agreed to make a video for the ASI and there was no way around explaining a film crew in the house! So I chose to tell the guys in very simple terms. I gave them the bare facts and said that I would answer any questions they had. They both knew I would never lie to them. They reacted exactly as I had anticipated. Matt presumed that I would be *old and grey* like Grandad before *things* changed.

Andrew was so very, very angry: he had an old shed where he mended and banded hurls, a welder and so on and for days all I heard was wood on wood, metal on metal and the air was blue with language. When he calmed down a bit and we chatted, it all poured out. He was angry that this had come to my door, especially with what I had already been through since childhood.

I am truly blessed to have an incredible relationship with both my sons. We never let a day close without connecting, saying I love you. We laugh and cry together and I tell that guys that tears and sadness will not kill us but keeping it in just might. We chat about everything and nothing is taboo. They have asked me what flowers I would like for my grave. They have also asked me to hang on till they are both earning and can afford good care for me and the toughest was one evening Andrew asked me if we had money to bury me (should anything happen suddenly). Well that broke my heart but like everything we worked on a plan. These guys have had to deal with some hard issues at a young age. They constantly challenge me and do not let me away with much. They encourage me to do what I am doing and tell me they are proud of me but most of all they inspire me to be the very best version of myself every single day.

In the early days I needed to speak to someone further along their journey but sadly the lady I met was so advanced in her dementia she could not hold a conversation and I was devastated. Since then I have made it known that I will travel to meet anyone newly diagnosed. Alzheimer's disease young or old is the same disease but the dynamics are very different for younger on-setters, probably still working who may have children at home and so on.

I have met with many and the difference it can make is incredible considering all it costs is the price of diesel and a coffee shared at a crucial time. To meet and chat with someone years into their journey can mean the difference of giving up or living as well as possible for as long as possible.

This is clearly the case especially if you hear 'get your affairs in order' at the same time as your diagnosis. Of course, it is important to put things in order but it is not helpful or conducive to hear this at diagnosis.

Life is never the same and it cannot ever be the same after diagnosis. There are new normals, sometimes even within the same day. I was encouraged early on to go on disability allowance – a big mistake. I thought professionals would know what was best for me, some did and some had not a clue. Apart from time on my hands, lack of finances, I now find myself not entitled to services and I am told that is because of my age. For example, I was refused a panic bracelet because I was under 65, even though my dementia advisor advised me to get one. No one with dementia should ever have to fight for care or support.

I found myself facing days of nothingness: friends were still working and there are only so many times you can hoover the house or walk the dogs. I badly needed to meet other people with younger-onset Alzheimer's disease, see what they were doing. So once I had told the guys, I was free to check out the Irish Dementia Working Group (IDWG) an advocacy group which is funded and supported by the ASI. I have to be honest here and say that I giggled at the thought of people with different dementias being part of a working group! How very wrong I was.

My need was greater than my scepticism and so I travelled to the Aisling Hotel in Dublin to meet with people running this group. It is no exaggeration to say my life changed for the better in joining this group. Entering that room that day it was a real turning point. I was immediately accepted without having to explain myself. I then met the most incredible people who have become dear friends. I gained a purpose, a sense of *can do*. I have done things in the last five and half years that I would never have dreamed possible.

I have been involved in all types of research, media work: I have spoken at conferences in Europe and I have had the privilege of completing two stages of the Camino to fundraise with the ASI. I have also sat on panels and participated in focus groups. I have met the most incredible, passionate people, all working hard to change the face and journey of dementia in Ireland. This is just some of what we do in the Working Group and it is not bad for people who many in society tend to write off!

I want to acknowledge that I could not have done any of this without the care, support, respect and encouragement from all in the Alzheimer Society of Ireland. I am so grateful to each and every one of you, as are my sons. When they hear what I am doing, it says that Mom is doing ok, that she's kicking ass and not just waiting to die.

I recently did the exact same assessment, the Wechsler Memory Scale-IV (WMS-IV) that I did six years ago, and I was so excited to see that on some of the tests I scored better than six years ago. I am told that the work I have been doing has challenged my brain in new and definitely different ways and this is part of the reason why I am so well today. I also believe that when you give, you get back so much more in return.

Life is getting more difficult and more challenging. This last year has seen Mr A take more ground but each time he does I try to work on it and think what can I do about this? Can I put a strategy in place and is this necessary in my life? Then I work on it or let it go.

Each day I start my prayer time with the serenity prayer and try to live by it. Then I close each day with thanks for the blessings I received during the day. I have peace in my heart and that makes all the difference. I have done all I can do for my future: I try to live in the moment since if I keep focussing on what is coming down the line that will rob me of today. I love, laugh, cry, enjoy a glass of wine. I am still me, still a Mom, a sister, an aunt, a friend, a child of God, a work colleague and I am still Kathy.

I was recently elected Chair of the Irish Dementia Working Group, a huge honour, in the last few years we have grown to four groups. There is much work to be done. We need a register to know what the real numbers of people living with dementia are. We need a post-diagnostic pathway for everyone – access to diagnosis should not just be dependent on where you live. We need dementia to be recognized as a long-term illness and we need individual appropriate care and support. This care should not just be for the person but for the family as well who are in the front line. We need early and timely diagnosis. We need the Assisted Decision-Making Capacity Act (ADMCA) implemented and not just written on paper. People under 65 must be entitled to services. At the moment they are not, and this is a disgrace when you consider we have up to 4000 people in Ireland with this young-onset dementia. In our Southern Irish Working

Group (of people with dementia) we have one person who is 40 years old. We need support for couples; support for children and teenagers; we need to keep on creating awareness; keep breaking down the stigma. This is just some of what needs to change.

Someone recently asked me to describe my life today. I have good days, bad days, foggy days and if I tell you I am discombobulated, watch out, you will know that it is a day I just need to be, so do not expect much from me. Most days are like walking through a minefield. I never know what skill or ability may disappear. Recently I got stuck putting on a wash; I just did not know what to do next. I cannot get into a lift with a black matt floor as I cannot convince myself that the floor is there, even though I tap it with my foot and touch it with my hand – it appears as if I will fall into a hole. If I do not focus on absolutely everything from getting out of bed till I go to bed at night something funny, silly or a little more serious can happen. Funny – I get out of the shower and wonder why my head is still full of shampoo! Silly – I am on the phone whilst madly looking for my phone all over the house! Serious – I forget to wear oven-mitts when I take a dish out of the oven. For me, to concentrate at this level is exhausting and sometimes it is hard to explain when it appears you have not done much.

Today was a good day: I finished this chapter, a miracle in itself. I worked on some research, remembered to cook dinner and did not have any mishaps!

CHAPTER 5

Informal caregivers of people with dementia

Introduction

This chapter addresses the topic of informal caregiving and dementia. In the first part, the meaning of informal care is clarified and differences between formal and informal care are identified. In this section, topics including motivation to care, hierarchies of care, differences between spouse and non-spouse caregivers and the changing tasks of dementia care are critically reviewed as are some well-known stress-coping models used to understand factors contributing to caregiver burden. The second part of the chapter advances to answer questions such as: who in Ireland are the informal caregivers; what care services do they provide; what type of income support do they receive from the government; why might caring be stressful and what factors influence the admission of people with dementia into long-term residential care? But first the focus is on a more general discussion of informal care.

Informal caregiving

Globally informal caregivers are the main source of support to people who need practical, personal and psychological assistance due to age, disability or long-term illnesses (Glendinning, 2018). Informal caregivers are also the main source of support to a person diagnosed with dementia (WHO, 2012; DOH, 2014) and may help to delay that person's admission to long-term residential care (Brodaty and Donkin, 2009). Informal caregivers are an extremely important resource for governments as they deliver a broad range of personal and social care services. These are services that if countries were to deliver formally would result in significant financial costs to governments (Zigante, 2018). To quantify their contribution, in a country like Ireland, informal caregivers are said to save the government €10 billion per year (Family Carers Ireland, 2019).

It is noted that in the EU, about 60% of the overall care required by people with dependency needs is delivered by informal caregivers (Genet et al., 2012) and EU estimates suggest that somewhere between 19 million to 125 million family members provide an average of twenty hours of care weekly to their family members (Glendinning, 2018). Considerable variation exists across Europe regarding the range and type of income supports available to informal caregivers (Zigante, 2018). There is also much variation regarding eligibility criteria for income support and the criteria used by countries to define who qualifies as an 'informal caregiver'.

Informal caregivers are generally family members[1] but occasionally friends, acquaintances or neighbours. The word 'informal' is somewhat of a misnomer as there is nothing particularly *informal* about what these caregivers do. However, the term is generally used to differentiate *informal* or *family caregivers* from *professional caregivers*, otherwise known as *formal caregivers*. This other category of caregiver constitutes an equally important group of service provider. However, the *formal caregiver* is a paid health service professional or care provider, employed to assist people who need support either at home in the community or in care homes or nursing homes. Although family members are traditionally unpaid, a common trend across many European countries today is to introduce cash payments to incentivize informal caregivers for the services they provide at home or to offer the care-recipient more choice. This means that the distinction between formal and informal and paid and unpaid caregiver is becoming increasingly blurred (Timonen, 2009; Zigante, 2018). Globally, women by far outnumber men in informal caregiving roles (Sharma, 2016; Verbakel et al., 2017).

---

[1] Informal caregivers are often referred to as family caregivers as they are generally family members. In this chapter, the two terms will be used interchangeably.

Informal caregivers can be any age, they can come from any socio-economic group, they may live with or apart from the person they are caring for and may also be gainfully employed. Informal caregivers help with everyday self-care activities or *activities of daily living* such as: dressing, grooming, using the bathroom/toileting activities. They also help with *instrumental activities of daily living* such as: managing transport, finance, shopping and phone calls. Some informal caregivers provide companionship and supervision and in the context of dementia, many become highly skilled at responding to *behaviours that challenge* such as repeated questioning, suspiciousness, hallucinations, delusions, agitation, aggression, apathy, depression and so on. Informal caregivers also help with other simple tasks that many of us take for granted like supporting the person transfer from a chair into bed. Some also provide nursing and technical support, as for example, incontinence management, catheter care, wound dressings, peg feeding and so on.

Conflicting policy agendas

Across many countries today, the pool of informal caregivers is diminishing and a growing concern across the EU and within member states is the future availability and willingness of women to provide informal care (Cahill, 2018b; Glendinning, 2018). Changing demographic trends including population ageing, changing migration patterns and changing family structures including smaller families, blended families and lone parenting, along with geographic mobility, are all factors likely to affect the future supply of informal caregivers. Changing female workforce trends, with higher rates of female participation in the paid labour market, will also affect the availability of informal caregivers, sometimes referred to as a 'reserve army of labour' (Twigg and Atkin, 1994).

In 2016, female labour market participation in EU28 averaged around 61% (Glendinning, 2018). However, this figure has risen more recently in line with the Europe 2020 Strategy. The latter aimed to ensure that three quarters of the population aged 20 to 64 years would be employed by 2020 (EDJN, 2019). Changing demographic trends along with the expected increase in women's labour market participation, will lead to a reduction in the availability of informal caregivers (Verbakel et al., 2017; Glendinning, 2018). There are therefore compelling reasons for governments to support informal caregivers to continue to work outside the home (Hoff et al., 2014; Larkin and Milne, 2017). Likewise there are important reasons for employers to promote carer-friendly workplaces by facilitating flexible working hours, flexible leave and by introducing measures to encourage informal caregivers to return to work after time off spent caring (Glendinning, 2018).

Dementia and hierarchies of care

Compared with other forms of caregiving, where the care role is often thrust on the informal caregiver unexpectedly, such as following a sudden stroke, the deterioration associated with dementia can be gradual and intermittent. Because of this, the dementia care role often unfolds incrementally without it ever being consciously adopted. Within families, a hierarchy of care is said to exist, where if a spouse is available, that spouse will adopt the informal caregiving role, but where there is no spouse, the role will devolve to an adult child, usually a daughter but sometimes a son or a daughter-in-law (Qureshi and Walker, 1989). Gender, kinship obligations, the relationship of the informal caregiver to the care-receiver and living arrangements can also determine who adopts the caring role (Pierce et al., 2017).

Motivation to care and differences between spouse and non-spouses

Informal or family caregivers most of whom are either spouses, adult children or adult children-in-law (Brodaty and Donkin, 2009), differ significantly in relation to their motivation and commitment to care. Marriage is usually considered the pre-eminent caring relationship and care within marriage is seen as a natural extension of marital vows (Pierce et al., 2017), whereas the injunction to care by adult children is generally not as intense or binding. Twigg and Atkin (1994) distinguish between these two categories of caregivers by referring to them as *engulfed carers* and *boundary setters*. According to them, *the engulfed carer* is often a spouse who subordinates her life for the person she cares for and allows caring to become the defining feature of her self-identity. In contrast, *boundary setters* are more likely to be adult children who can distance themselves from their loved ones and place greater value on their own autonomy creating time for their own interests.

Whereas spouses often identify love, reciprocity and compassion as reasons for caring, reasons cited by adult children include duty/gendered kinship obligations, geographical proximity, labour market positioning and the lack of availability of other family members (Ungerson, 1987; Cahill, 1997, 1999; Pierce et al., 2017). In other words, often a daughter or daughter-in-law adopts the caring role because she feels obliged to do so because of her gender, or lives nearby or is not gainfully employed and has no child-care or other legitimate commitments to exempt herself. Essentially this means that the informal caregiver may be the weakest link in the kinship network. Understanding what motivates family members to become informal caregivers is important as is choice (Pertl et al., 2019) as when caregiving roles are taken on reluctantly, this may have important ramifications for the quality of care and quality of life of both the caregiver and care-receiver (Cahill, 1999).

The tasks of dementia care

Early stage

Dementia care can be hard physical and emotional labour and it is often associated with long hours spent delivering care services (Brodaty and Donkin, 2009). Informal caregiving is *labour* and *love*: it is *caring about* as well as *caring for* and the *caring for* services are often diverse, unpredictable and progressive (Pierce et al., 2017). They can change daily and in accordance with the dementia sub-type, the presence of other co-morbidities and the disease severity. For example, in the early stages, the only help required may be that of supporting a relative to come to terms with the diagnosis and with some of the losses associated (Pierce et al., 2017). Assistance may also be needed in decision-making about who to tell and what to say about the diagnosis; in the participation of making or updating a will or an Enduring Power of Attorney (EPA) and with memory problems such as regular reminders about when to take medication and so on. This may sound simple, but the reality is that providing practical and emotional support whilst simultaneously promoting a loved one's dignity, personhood, humanity, independence and autonomy can be challenging, especially if the person lacks insight and is unwilling or unable to acknowledge their deficits. Dementia can impair insight and judgment, but it does not impair the natural desire we all have to remain independent and be in control of our lives. Accordingly, the provision of personalized service supports often demands creative subtle and sensitive approaches.

Moderate stage

In the more moderate stages of dementia, common concerns include safety and self-neglect. The person may be prone to engage in potentially dangerous activities or may forget to eat regularly or neglect their hygiene. Accordingly, considerable support may be needed in the careful watching over a loved one and in providing assistance with grooming, dressing, showering and toileting. What is critically important here is knowing the level of support that is acceptable to the person and providing that support in a dignity-enhancing way. Resistance to caregiver support is not uncommon and efforts by the informal caregiver to help that person, especially with personal hygiene may culminate in episodes of agitation and aggression (Cahill and Shapiro, 1993).

Agitation and low to moderate levels of aggression along with other *behaviours that challenge* such as repeated questioning, suspiciousness, paranoia, delusions, hallucinations, apathy, wandering, hoarding, anxiety, depression and disinhibition, cause informal caregivers much distress and are likely to come to the fore as dementia progresses (Benoit, 2006). Commonly referred to as the *behavioural and psychological symptoms of dementia*, the jury is out on the exact cause of these behaviours. However, the reality is that probably a complex interplay of biological, psychological, environmental and social factors causes the behaviours (Brooker and Latham, 2016).

It is also important to remember that *behaviours that challenge* never occur in isolation but rather are part of a dynamic process involving the individual, the environment and the caregiver (Byrne et al., 2006). Rather than being seen as symptoms of a pathology, often these behaviours are best understood as attempts to communicate some unmet need (Stokes, 2011). No matter what precipitates these behaviours, they can have a profound impact on the informal caregiver. A recent review (Cheng, 2017) has shown that agitation, aggression and disinhibition are considered most disturbing for informal caregivers. This is partly because they exacerbate difficulties in other domains like *activities of daily living* but also, as in the case of rarer forms of dementias, like frontotemporal, because of the care-recipients' insensitivity to the feelings of others: an insensitivity generally caused by the dementia.

Responses to *behaviours that challenge* should first involve the identification of the cause of the behaviour with consideration given to the emotions underpinning the behaviour (Zarit and Zarit, 2007). In other words, informal caregivers should first look for the trigger factor that leads to the behaviour, analyse the behaviour and review the consequences of how the behaviour has been responded to, including the extent to which that response may have unwittingly reinforced the behaviour (Zarit and Zarit, 2007; Krishnamoorthy and Anderson, 2011). Antipsychotic medication, although often used to address these *behaviours,* can produce adverse and at the extreme catastrophic reactions (Banerjee, 2009) and should only ever be used as a last resort.

Advanced stage

At the more advanced stages of dementia, the support provided by the informal caregiver is likely to extend around the clock and will include careful supervision, coordinating care, offering emotional encouragement, providing some form of psychosocial stimulation and ongoing monitoring. With more severe dementia the person can have more extensive memory loss problems, although fewer *behaviours that challenge*, limited or no mobility and difficulty with eating and swallowing. The person may also be incontinent of bowel and bladder (Newhouse and Lasek, 2006) and may have screaming episodes (Eastwood, 1994). Since the person can usually no longer converse fluently, the informal caregiver may have to wear a 'detective hat' always attempting to understand the meaning behind the behaviour.

Connecting into the individual's non-verbal communication and working with the person's senses, such as hearing, touch, or sight may provide some solace. Slow hand massage, listening to music or the sounds from nature, smiles, gestures and speaking or singing softly may help to relax the anxious person. Contrary to some peoples' thinking, the person with an advanced dementia, although usually deficient in language skills, is not 'gone' or 'socially dead' and is not just a body to be washed cleaned and fed (Lindemann, 2014). That person is still a *human being* that needs ongoing human contact and personalized care and support. And although the individual may no longer be able to recognize familiar faces by name or in the narrow cognitive sense, recognition of voice, touch, or scent may remain well into the more advanced stages of dementia.

Caregiving burden and dementia care

Providing dementia care can be extremely demanding and caring may adversely affect a family caregiver's own physical and emotional health (Pinquart and Sörensen, 2003; Berglund et al., 2015). Numerous studies have shown that caring for a person with dementia is more stressful than caring for someone with a physical disability (Brodaty and Donkin,

2009; Teahan et al., 2020). In the USA, Fortinsky et al. (2013) have shown that informal caregivers of people diagnosed with dementia have higher rates of anxiety and clinical depression and experience poorer emotional health compared with non-caregivers (Fortinsky et al., 2013). In Australia, Brodaty et al. (2009) have shown that family caregivers of people with dementia are at increased risk of developing cardiovascular problems, have lower immunity, higher levels of chronic diseases, more doctor visits and have a greater likelihood of smoking, drinking alcohol and experiencing poor sleep patterns. One meta-analysis found that family caregivers of people with dementia experienced more severe depression and physical illnesses and were more stressed than non-dementia caregivers (Pinquart and Sörensen, 2003)

Caregiver burden and stress-coping models

Different models of factors leading to caregiver burden have been identified in the literature (Poulshock and Deimling, 1984; Pearlin et al., 1990; Gaugler et al., 2000). Much of this earlier literature has drawn on stress-coping models to understand the dynamics of informal care, including the key stressors and the key coping strategies required to help reduce caregiver burden (Cahill, 1997). In this early literature, caregiver burden was defined as: 'the physical, psychological, emotional, social and financial problems that can be experienced by family members caring for impaired older adults' (George and Gwyther, 1986, p. 253) and great effort was invested into examining the correlates of burden and into measuring *objective* versus *subjective burden*. Likewise, considerable effort was invested into identifying coping strategies that could be used to reduce caregiver burden (Lazarus and Folkman, 1984).

Subjective and objective burden

The burden or stress of caregiving has often been described as both subjective and objective. *Subjective burden* refers to a carer's own assessment of the harmful impact the care role has on them and their emotional reaction to stressors (Matsuda, 1999). In contrast *objective burden* refers to the costs of caring, such as time spent providing care and time lost from work due to caring responsibilities (Wolfs et al., 2012). The well-known and easy to administer scale for measuring *subjective caregiver burden*, (Zarit et al., 1980) and its shortened twelve item version, captures caregivers' own subjective appraisal of how caring affects their lives. The items on the scale include: carer's health, their psychological well-being, finances, social life and the nature of the relationship between the caregiver and the person living with dementia.

In Pearlin et al.'s stress-coping model (1990), a distinction is made between *primary stressors* and *secondary stressors*. *Primary stressors* refer to characteristics of the person living with dementia. These include the cognitive impairment, behaviours that challenge and dependency levels. *Secondary stressors* refer to the overflow of care activities into other areas of the caregiver's life. Examples here include how care activities impact on finance, work and the carer's social world. In this model, coping strategies, like seeking social support through availing of educational interventions (see Chapter 3), can reduce caregiver stress and improve caregiver health.

In the well cited, Poulshock and Deimling model (1984), dementia leads to a burden of care that manifests as strain and can be increased or decreased in different ways. Like other models, the Poulshock and Deimling model also differentiates between *primary* and *secondary stressors*. *Primary stressors* arise mainly from the needs of the person who has dementia and how these needs determine the level of care required. *Primary stressors* can produce *secondary stressors* that include role strain and intrapsychic strain or a reduction in the positive elements of self, including role captivity. This international literature has shown that caregiver stress[2] is multidimensional. Providing care can adversely affect a family caregiver's physical health: it can contribute to financial hardship, social isolation and psychological morbidity (Brodaty and Donkin, 2009).

Now having briefly reviewed some key findings from the international literature on stress-coping models, the next section of the chapter looks at the Irish context of dementia care and specifically at the role of informal caregivers in Ireland. How many Irish family members deliver informal care

---

2   It should be remembered that there is also a growing body of literature on the topic of caregiver gratification and caregiver resilience (Teehan et al, 2018).

to their relatives living with dementia? How much help do these informal caregivers receive from the government and from other family members? What are the challenges confronting informal caregivers and what causes them most distress? The section to follow addresses these questions.

Informal caregiving to a person with dementia in Ireland

Although many of the demographic changes discussed in this chapter are already being witnessed in Ireland, women's labour market participation is still low by European standards but this trend is likely to change over coming years (Bercholz and Fitzgerald, 2016; Keogh et al., 2019). Any future reduction in the supply of informal caregivers in Ireland, for reasons such as changes in female labour market participation, changes in family size and structure, changing migration patterns, changes in motivation to care and so on, will have serious implications for the care of people who have dementia (Walsh et al., 2019). According to some, this issue – the future decline in the availability of informal caregivers in Ireland – has not been given sufficient political attention (Daly, 2018) and there is a need for more workplace flexibility in Ireland to support informal carers who want to and need to work outside the home.

As mentioned, in Ireland, about 30,000 men and women who have dementia live at home in the community, where most receive support from informal caregivers, mainly family members (Pierse et al., 2017). Although Census data on informal caregivers exists along with other caregiver data[3] (Pierce et al., 2017), there is no valid and reliable data on how many of these informal caregivers deliver dementia care. Recent estimates[4] suggest that there are about 60,000 informal caregivers who support their relatives with dementia to live at home. This figure may be an under-estimate since many family caregivers remain heavily committed to dementia care

---

3   Based on the 2016 Census there were 195,262 informal caregivers in Ireland.
4   This figure has been estimated by extrapolating from the Enhancing Care in Alzheimer's Disease (ECAD) study, which found that community-dwelling people with dementia had an average of 1.7 caregivers (Gillespie et al., 2013).

even after their relative has moved into a nursing home or a residential care setting (Brennan et al., 2017).

While the Government purports to support informal caregivers in Ireland (DOH, 2014), the reality is that home care is provided on a non-statutory basis. Accordingly, home care is essentially family care and family care is usually care provided by women, occasionally supplemented by government services (Pertl et al., 2019). In this way, home care in Ireland differs from many of the Nordic countries where elder care is a state, regional or municipality responsibility rather than a family responsibility. In these other countries family caregivers generally play a less intensive role in home care provision (Verbakel et al., 2017). There is still no legislative basis for home care services in Ireland and an incongruence in government policy that claims to favour home care over long-term residential care (Hanly and Sheerin, 2017), yet apportions a significantly larger percentage of the health budget to long-term residential care services.

In Ireland nearly half (48%) of the €1.69 billion annual cost of dementia care can be attributed to the opportunity costs (income opportunities foregone) of informal caregivers, whilst 43% of costs are attributable to residential care (Connolly et al., 2014). As noted by Connolly et al. (2014), in 2010, family and friends delivered an estimated eighty-one million hours of care to people with dementia, saving the Irish government an estimated €807 million. These informal caregivers, mostly women are the *experts*. They are often the most important resource for people diagnosed with dementia (Livingston et al., 2017). In Ireland informal caregivers want to provide care but they also want recognition from the State for the very significant contribution they make (O'Shea, 2003).

Government support of informal caregivers of persons living with dementia

Although no legislation exists for home care services in Ireland, the country has supposedly generous legislation in place to support informal caregivers take time off work to care (Family Carers Ireland,

2017). A number of measures exist that make cash payments available to carers for their caregiving work (Daly, 2018). For eligible caregivers, a means tested Carer's Allowance or a non-means tested Carer's Benefit is available. The Carer's Allowance is available to those who provide full-time care and who broadly speaking have not been in gainful employment prior to adopting the primary care role. The Carer's Benefit is available to those who have been in gainful employment but who must stop paid work to care full time. Underpinning these income supports is the Carer's Leave act: legislation that entitles informal caregivers to unpaid leave, to provide full time care to a dependent for a maximum period of 104 months. There is widespread lack of knowledge amongst Irish informal caregivers about income support entitlements for caring and a poor take up on such supports. For example, as at July 2018, only 1.3% of all informal caregivers in Ireland were in receipt of the Carer's Benefit (Cahill, 2018b).

One advantage of the Carer's Allowance is that it entitles the caregiver to a household care package that includes a gas or electricity allowance, a free TV licence and in certain instances a small travel allowance. However, a requirement is that the informal caregiver must be co-resident with the care-recipient. Full-time informal caregivers in Ireland are also eligible for a 'Carer Support Grant' that pays about €2,000 per annum and can be used according to need. In addition, tax credits are available for the spouse or partner of full-time caregivers if employed in the labour market.

Home support services

Most Irish people who have dementia want to live at home for as long as possible (Keogh et al., 2019) and formal home-based supports are also available to assist informal caregivers continue to provide home care (Hanly and Sheerin, 2017). Formal home-based supports now called Home Support Services consist mainly of home help and home care packages. Home help focuses mainly on personal care such as washing, showering, mobility, hygiene or help at mealtime. It also focuses on domestic duties such as lighting the fire or bringing the fuel in or cleaning the person's bathroom or bedroom. In contrast home care packages (HCPS) are services that are often individualized and designed to help an older person stay at home (Keogh et al., 2018a). In practice however, these services are similar to home help services except they provide more hours of support. Traditionally the provision of hours under HCPS schemes was restricted, in fact rationed with an emphasis on task-oriented care (Dempsey et al., 2016).

More recently and as part of the implementation of the NDS, new dementia-specific intensive home care packages (IHCP) were delivered to a select group of people diagnosed with dementia. Compared with usual home supports, this new scheme provided higher levels of funding and was intended to provide a wider range of flexible personalized supports to informal caregivers (Keogh et al., 2018a). Service supports available included: personal care, supervision and maintenance of personhood and life roles, nursing or allied health interventions, aids and appliances and respite support services including in-home respite and overnight care. As of the end of February 2018, 309 people diagnosed with dementia or 1% of all community-dwellers, had benefitted from these IHCP (HSE, 2018). When first introduced, the allocation of IHCP was linked to delayed hospital discharge and the new bundle of IHCP was used to address overcrowding problems in hospitals (ASI, 2019).

An evaluation of this new service revealed that IHCP can help people with dementia, even those with significant levels of disability and cognitive impairment, to stay at home for longer. Other preliminary findings showed that those receiving IHCP were less likely to be admitted to residential care than other similarly dependent people. It was concluded that IHCP reflected value for money, especially for people on the boundaries between community and residential care (Keogh et al., 2018b).

There is enormous demand for HCPS in Ireland and although figures on the numbers of people with dementia currently wait-listed for this service are not available, it is estimated that an additional 10,000 home care packages will be required for older people over the next decade (Sage, 2018). The recent health service capacity review also suggests that because of population ageing, the demand for both HCPS and IHCP will increase by about 70% over the next decade (PA Consulting, 2018).

Caregiver burden in Ireland

Like in other countries, most Irish informal caregivers who support their relatives living with dementia, experience high levels of stress. Two recent studies have helped to shed new light on the stress of dementia care and the way in which caring affects family caregivers' health and well-being. One of these (Lafferty et al., 2016) involved a secondary analysis of a sample of 485 family caregivers who were providing dementia care. This sample was drawn from a national register of 4000 family carers of older people, all in receipt of the Carer's Allowance (Lafferty et al., 2014). The carers were mostly women (73%) and the majority were adult children. Three quarters lived with their relative who had dementia. Just under half (47%) reported they experienced moderate to severe caregiver burden and just over half (51%) were considered at risk for developing clinical depression. A little over one third of these caregivers rated their health as only fair or poor. Findings showed that the majority of these informal caregivers spent more than eighty hours a week caring and about 10% were also doing paid work outside the home. Two thirds were aged less than 65 years, a finding that suggests that many were probably 'women in the middle' caring for children, spouses and elderly parents. The tasks undertaken by these caregivers included housework (85%), bathing and showering (71%), dressing and undressing (54%) walking (47%) cutting and help with eating food (46%) and toileting (39%). Only about one third of these family carers reported they received training to help them care for their relative who had dementia.

These findings regarding the stress of dementia care were re-echoed by Brennan et al., (2017) in a study that looked at the daily lives of spouse caregivers supporting their relatives with dementia. In this study, most spouses were wives and three quarters were aged over 65 years. Results showed that more than three quarters spent all their waking hours caregiving, and many remained fully committed to the care role even after their relative was admitted to long-term residential care. Close to half (42%) of these spouses received no help from other family members or friends in the month prior to the research interview. Only about 50% received state or private home care supports. Some caregivers were working at the time of their spouses' diagnosis and about 15% had to stop work to care. Not surprisingly *behaviours that challenge* such as agitation, aggression, anxiety and irritability caused spouse caregivers most distress. In keeping with the literature, findings also demonstrated that family caregivers' own health was not good. The majority (70%) experienced at least two chronic health problems and took prescribed medicine for their illnesses. Most had also visited a health care professional at least once in the month prior to interview. More than one third of these spouse caregivers were diagnosed with depression.

Since the publication of this Irish report, further analysis of the De-Stress data has shown that age, gender and place of residence were factors associated with the cessation of informal care. A person whose informal caregiver was aged 70 and over was more likely to be admitted to long-term residential care compared with those whose caregiver was aged under 60 years. Likewise, having a male informal caregiver increased the likelihood of nursing home admission at one-year follow-up. Interestingly living in a rural area reduced the risk of nursing home care admission. Other factors identified as determining nursing home admission included psychosis and greater impairments in activities of daily living (Walsh et al., 2019).

Conclusions

Written against the backdrop of the international literature, this chapter has shown that caring for a relative with dementia can be labour-intensive and physically and emotionally demanding. Caregiving is a gendered issue and the tasks associated with informal caregiving are diverse, unpredictable and can extend around the clock accumulating over time to the point where the caregiver's own physical and mental health may deteriorate. The chapter has also shown that informal caregiving entails both *caring for* and *caring about*: it is an *activity* along with an *identity* that is both *personal* and *political*. Regrettably governments often emphasize the *caring about* aspect of care without giving due attention to the hard, physical *caring for* aspects of the care role.

Two recent Irish studies reviewed in this chapter have also shed new light on the tasks of dementia care, the type of caregiver burden experienced and the limited supports received by spouses and adult children whilst attempting to provide dementia care. These studies have shown that in the context of dementia, informal caregivers of whom there are about 60,000, save the government sizeable sums of money, but receive little financial support or home care services for the unpaid services they deliver. While there may be an expectation that family members should provide care to their frail older relatives, changing demographics and changing ideologies may impact on the future availability and capacity of women to deliver these services.

There is a need for more realistic investment in home care services for people who have dementia and wish to continue to live at home. If government policy is truly committed to home-based care, then the funding system must change to reflect a more visionary, flexible and personalized form of home-based care. Caregiving needs to be seen as a continuum and a diverse range of coordinated integrated care services needs to be developed that will help to reduce the burden of care currently experienced by informal caregivers. The development of a new continuum of care model and the future recalibration of care will be discussed in Chapter 7 of this book. But next to a chapter which brings the focus back to the individual who is living with dementia.

CHAPTER 6

Personhood, autonomy capacity and decision-making

Introduction

In this chapter attention returns to the person living with dementia and to what informal and formal caregivers, family members and friends can do to promote that person's personhood, independence, autonomy and dignity and help the individual enjoy a good quality of life. Several misunderstandings about dementia prevail in society and there is a tendency for the public to regard all dementias as the same and sometimes to consider a diagnosis as a death sentence, when in fact there is huge diversity in presentations of dementia and in how people experience their symptoms. There is also much diversity in the degree of severity experienced in cognitive impairments and in the behaviour, actions, mood, abilities and disabilities of people diagnosed (Taylor, 2008). Indeed day-by-day, minute by minute, the individual's subjective experience and behaviour is liable to fluctuate.

We live in a hyper-cognitive world where an undue emphasis is often placed on smart thinking, rationality and economic productivity (Post, 2000; Hughes, 2014). A person whose mind is no longer razor-sharp may be made to feel inferior by others and may be marginalized, ridiculed, dismissed and excluded from mainstream society (Mental Health Foundation, 2016). A nihilist discourse of tragedy doom and gloom about dementia can also prevail (George, 2010; Gilmour and Brannelly, 2010; Gove et al., 2015). Ageism is rife in society and dementia is often equated with old age and with end-stage Alzheimer's disease. The latter is seen primarily as a terminal illness or fatal with no hope, no cure; a progressive and irreversible cognitive brain disorder, that 'robs' the individual of their humanity and ultimately leads to an untimely death.

Words are powerful; it is not just about the words, but it is about how we view the person when we describe them with these words that matters and the tragedy discourse does nothing to promote the dignity and humanity of the individual. Irrespective of the severity of the condition the person living with dementia will always remain an emotional thinking human being that must be respected and treated with dignity and not relegated to the position of a *conversationlist ghost* (Davis and Pope, 2010) where the person is continuously ignored and left out of conversation.

The *negative positioning* (Sabat, 2019) can also shape and inform our daily interactions with the person diagnosed and can influence policy responses including how community and residential care service supports are designed and delivered. Dementia can be an extremely frightening condition and it may be all the more terrifying, if negative and prejudicial attitudes are inadvertently communicated to the person experiencing the symptoms. Through our behaviour, language and interactions all of us can play a key role in either supporting or hindering the person's experience of dementia.

Understanding of dementia over time

Our thinking and how we talk about dementia have also changed significantly over time. For example, historically in Ireland, when an older person developed dementia it was seen as a normal part of ageing and the confused older person was often described as having 'a bit of senility'. Expressions like *he has become doddery, she is away with the fairies* and in *cloud cuckoo land* were often used to describe that person's cognitive and memory loss problems and changed behaviour. Considered stigmatizing (Nolan et al., 2006), dementia remained somewhat invisible and for reasons including ignorance, shame, embarrassment and fear, people tended not to talk about it. The individual was often silenced, set apart from others, sometimes hidden and often seen as a lesser rather than a fuller member of society. Once diagnosed, that person's right to independent decision-making was often automatically removed (Nuffield Council on Bioethics, 2009; O'Connor and Purves, 2009; Cahill, 2018a) and their lived experiences were disregarded.

Then when the condition progressed and memory, cognitive, behavioural and social functioning became significantly impaired, the person was in the 1950s and 1960s, often transferred from home into a nursing home. There, in a hospital-style nightingale ward or worse still a locked psychiatric institution, an emphasis was placed on custodial, clinical, technical care and on chemical and physical restraints. Advances in medicine, psychiatry, bioethics, psychology, nursing, sociology, disability and dementia studies have changed this way of thinking (Bartlett and O'Connor, 2007; Innes, 2009; WHO, 2012) and today dementia is no longer seen as a normal part of ageing but rather it is a syndrome caused by one of many underlying diseases. The reframing of 'personhood', a concept that will be discussed later in this chapter, also has a major impact on how dementia care services are now being developed and delivered.

Kahn's contribution to a shift in thinking about senility and dementia

Although rarely acknowledged, a founding father likely to have influenced this fundamental shift in thinking about dementia was the US academic Robert Kahn (Steve Zarit, personal communication, January 2019). A pioneer of Geriatric Psychology, attached to the university of Chicago and writing about senility[1] in the 1970's, Kahn was one of the first to critique the biomedical model and in particular mental health care services, described by him as *nihilistic* and *custodial* (Kahn, 1975).

---

1   Writing in the 70's Kahn used the term senility to refer to dementia.

For Kahn, custodialism reflected a therapeutic nihilism where 'senile patients' were seen as dangerous, unpredictable and viewed as different from 'normal' people. Because of this, they were set apart and required long-term care in highly controlled settings. Kahn critiqued what he referred to as hierarchical structures in these controlled mental health settings since within such environments: 'the patient [was] occupying the lowest status position in the hierarchy' (p. 27) and care often focused on *detention* and *safeguarding* that could further disable the individual.

Kahn was ahead of his time in demonstrating how interventions can be both harmful and helpful to those diagnosed with 'senility'. He claimed that minimal intervention or the least disruptive supports provided in regular domestic settings were preferable to therapeutic intervention. His appeal was for innovation in mental health services and for interventions that might empower, promote autonomy and return to the person a sense of control. For Kahn, the very act of being supported could increase 'impairment' because of loss of control and 'infantalization'. Interestingly it was at the US Philadelphia Geriatric Centre where Kahn first introduced the concept of *excess disability* – or disability embedded in the social world rather than in the brain; a phenomenon he claimed arose as a consequence of custodial or institutional care.

Most importantly Kahn emphasized the importance of viewing 'senility' as a psycho-social-biological phenomenon. In this context, he was probably one of the first to argue that although we cannot address the biological or the neurophysiological aspects of senility such as halt the symptoms, we can manipulate the physical and psychosocial environment including organizational structures to support the person. So, for example, by exposing the individual to a richer more stimulating environment, a person's excess disabilities could be reduced. Whilst Kahn's legacy to the field of mental health and dementia services has been enormous, his focus was on systems and structure failures which led to excess disability rather than on personhood and autonomy, concepts which were to be later unpicked almost exhaustively by other writers likely to have built on Kahn's ground-breaking work.

Kitwood's contribution and the emergence of personhood as a key concept in dementia care

Since Kahn's time, much has been written about the value of applying a social and biopsychosocial lens to help deconstruct dementia (see, e.g., Bond, 2001; Sabat 2001, 2014; Sabat et al., 2011). A burgeoning body of literature has also been developed on the topic of personhood (see, e.g., Hung and Chaudhury, 2011; Bartlett and O'Connor, 2007; Dewing, 2008; Murray and Boyd, 2009; Bartlett and O'Connor, 2010; Quinn, 2010; McCormack et al., 2012; Flynn and Arstein-Kerslake, 2014; Gilleard and Higgs, 2016; Hennelly et al., 2018, 2019 and Bosco et al., 2019). Defined by Kitwood (1997a, p. 8) as: 'That status bestowed on one human being by another in the context of relationships and social standing it implies recognition, respect and trust', Kitwood's definition of personhood overturned the original Cartesian view that personhood was cognitively based or that personhood was located in the mind.

Kitwood was a UK-based clinical psychologist who had worked for years in dementia care settings. His deconstruction of personhood in the late 1990's was revolutionary since traditional understandings of personhood had been heavily embedded in philosophical assumptions held about cognitive ability, rational thinking and consciousness (Blackburn, 2005; Bartlett and O'Connor, 2010) and on the assumption that the *thinking mind* was both the site of and a prerequisite for personhood. In other words, a person was only a person because they had the capacity for rational thinking. Over the years, questions were raised about the association between personhood and rationality including, for example, if the individual can be the same person despite significant memory loss (Cohen and Eisdorfer, 1986). Indeed, in a controversial piece of work published in 1988, an appallingly reductionist view of personhood was espoused. In this work, people with severe dementia were compared to animals; severe dementia was believed to destroy memories and it also caused the erosion of personhood (Brock, 1988). Such comparisons have more recently been reiterated in the literature (see, e.g., Svendsen et al., 2018).

Kitwood (1997a) challenged such inhumane perspectives by placing an emphasis on the relational aspects of personhood and the role others played in preserving it. A former clergyman and humanitarian in his outlook, he was greatly disillusioned by the services he saw delivered in traditional care settings. Kitwood (1997a) labelled this, the *old culture of care* which for him was oppressive, technical and based on hierarchical care relationships and not on values of respect, trust and communication. He argued that the decline associated with dementia occurred not only because of the diseased brain (a biomedical explanation) but also because of an erosion of personhood caused by a 'malignant social psychology' (p. 19) (a biopsychosocial explanation) that dehumanized the individual. In this way, Kitwood's theorizing of dementia and personhood displaced the biomedical model.

Kitwood and Bredin (1992) argued that personhood was dynamic: it was created and re-created in social relationships and reinstated and sustained by others. Best practice was about preserving personhood, promoting confidence and dignity in the individual, addressing that person's psychological needs and recognizing that biographical, environmental, social and cultural factors influenced the person's experience of dementia (Kitwood, 1993a). In his view even people with a very severe dementia could still have their personhood maintained through dignity-enhancing person-centred relationships and through having their psychological needs addressed. He wrote:

> In dementia the inner sense of stability and security, held in place through memory and judgment, is vanishing to nothing. Now personhood can only be guaranteed, replenished and sustained through what others provide. And as the neuropathology advances, reducing individual capability, the need for that 'person work' will grow more, not less. This is the fundamental challenge for good dementia care. (Kitwood, 1993a, p. 545)

Kitwood was deeply committed to improving dementia care. What concerned him a lot was how slowly practice was changing and how long it was taking for dementia care to be humanized. Too often he claimed people were pathologized and treated as non-persons. He wrote: 'The old culture generally denied the existence of psychological need in people with dementia, or blanked it out with tranquillizing medication.' (Kitwood, 1997a, p. 135). His contributions to re-conceptualizing dementia and reframing personhood (Kitwood, 1990, 1993a, b, 1995, 1997a, b) have been most valuable and have had a very profound influence on contemporary theoretical understandings. Indeed today, personhood is considered to be the cornerstone of best practice and a critical component of person-centred care for the individual living with dementia (Hennelly et al., 2019).

Personhood and autonomy

So far in this chapter, personhood has been discussed in the context of dementia, but central to our understanding of personhood is autonomy (McCormack, 2001; Boyle, 2008; O'Connor et al., 2009; Murphy and Welford, 2012; OECD, 2015; Hennelly et al., 2019): a concept that can be defined in many different ways (see, e.g., Boyle, 2008). There is some consensus in the literature that autonomy refers to self-determination (O'Connor et al., 2009) and to an understanding that human beings must be respected and allowed to direct their lives in accordance with their own personal beliefs, values and preferences (HIQA, 2016). Choice and control are therefore central tenets of autonomy (O'Shea et al., 2019), a concept that is also linked to 'dignity', (Nordenfelt, 2004; CRPD, 2006; Nuffield Council on Bioethics, 2009) and to 'privacy' (Cahill, 2018a). In gerontological research, autonomy is also considered a critical component of older peoples' quality of life (Kane, 2001; Boyle, 2008; Nuffield Council on Bioethics, 2009; Murphy and Welford, 2012; Hughes, 2014; Smebye et al., 2016; Donnelly et al., 2018).

But in discussions about autonomy and dementia, the elephant in the room so to speak is *capacity* – an important concept, integral to our understanding of autonomy. In fact, some would argue that in discussions about autonomy, an unprecedented focus is placed on capacity to the detriment of its other attributes (Nuffield Council on Bioethics, 2009; O'Connor et al.,

2009; Donnelly et al., 2018). Capacity is a complex multidimensional concept[2]: it refers to both (i) mental capacity, the ability to engage in rational decision-making, and (ii) legal capacity or the legal right to make decisions.

Mental capacity is determined by a health service professional and typically requires the person to understand, retain, use and weigh up information and options in order to make and communicate a decision. Legal capacity in contrast, is typically determined by a lawyer (O'Connor and Purves, 2009) and refers to the recognition that a person is both the holder and executor of legal rights (Flynn, 2018). While mental capacity and legal capacity are inter-related, mental capacity is not a prerequisite for legal capacity. A person can have diminished mental capacity but is still within their rights to exercise their legal capacity (Flynn, 2018). For example, a person may be disorientated in time and place and may no longer display rational thinking, but that person still retains a legal right to refuse admission to a nursing home or refuse to have a health care assistant visit their home.

Similar to metaphysical concepts of personhood that place an undue emphasis on rationality (Hennelly et al., 2019), traditional accounts of autonomy have tended to define it along cognitive lines with the assumption that to exercise autonomy a person must have capacity for rational thinking (Nuffield Council on Bioethics, 2009). Since dementia impaired rationality, a diagnosis was often used as grounds to deny a person's autonomy rights (Flynn, 2018). So, in hospitals or care settings, a type of paternalism often occurred where family members were routinely seen as substitute decision-makers and asked to sign consent forms to enable staff to proceed with interventions. This was often done without first attempting to gain consent from the individual or to assess that person's capacity to make a particular decision. In many countries including Ireland, the law supported this type of paternalism with substitute rather than supportive models of decision-making in evidence (AE, 2012; Flynn, 2018). In other words, the denial of legal capacity was often imposed as a direct consequence of poor performance on a mental capacity assessment (Sabat, 2005; Flynn, 2018).

---

2   The concept also includes testamentary capacity or a person's legal and mental ability to make a will.

More recently, this conventional and restrictive thinking about autonomy has been challenged (see, e.g., Pullman, 1999; McCormack, 2001; Kittay, 2007; Nuffield Council on Bioethics, 2009; O'Connor and Purves, 2009; Hughes, 2011, 2014; Smebye et al., 2015; Donnelly et al., 2018) and nowadays a broader more holistic understanding is held in most jurisdictions. Proponents of this more nuanced understanding of autonomy argue that, although a person may have impaired capacity and may have lost the rational ability to formulate and communicate a decision, they can still have 'relational autonomy'[3] and can generally be supported to express their views and preferences and to value one thing over another. Heggestad et al. (2015, p. 837) note that: 'Relational autonomy makes it possible to confirm individuals with dementia as equal human beings, despite their cognitive impairments.' This approach takes cognizance of the fact that capacity can fluctuate and must always be regarded as being: (i) time, (ii) circumstance and (iii) decision-specific (Tilse et al., 2009). In Ireland this broader approach to understanding capacity and respecting autonomy, often referred to as the functional approach, is well embedded in the Assisted Decision-Making (Capacity) Act (ADMCA, 2015).

The Assisted Decision-Making Capacity Act (2015)

The Assisted Decision-Making Capacity Act (ADMCA) was first signed into law in Ireland in December 2015. It was part of a series of law reforms introduced to enable Ireland to ratify the UN Convention on the Rights of Persons with Disability (CRPD, 2006). For an excellent overview of the ADMCA, see Donnelly, 2019. The ADMCA asserts that in Ireland a person shall not be regarded as being unable to engage in decision-making, unless all practical steps have first been taken and have

---

[3] An approach that recognizes that respect for autonomy must involve others being proactive in promoting that person's autonomy (Nuffield Council on Bioethics, 2009).

failed to help that person to do so. The guiding principles underpinning the ADMCA are the presumption of capacity and the requirement that a person should be given all possible support available to make their own decisions. In this way the Act enshrines a legal right to autonomy for a person whose mental capacity may be compromised (Donnelly, 2019). Although regrettably the Act has still not fully come into effect[4] when it does, it will have significant ramifications for many people including those living with dementia.

Tiered levels of decision-making

The ADMCA provides a statutory framework for different levels of decision-making appropriate to the person's needs. At the lowest level, the person whose decision-making capacity is currently or may soon *come into question*, can appoint an assistant-decision-maker (ADM) to help them acquire relevant and necessary information, consider options, help to communicate a decision and ensure the person's decision is implemented (Flynn, 2018). The appointment of an ADM can be made in relation to decisions about personal welfare such as health care and/or property and affairs and the person can nominate one or several ADMs. Importantly at the time of appointing the ADM, the person must be able to understand the nature and consequences of their decisions in the context of all available choices (Donnelly, 2019).

At the next level, the person may legally appoint a co-decision-maker (CDM), who jointly engages with them in decision-making. The appointment of a CDM is a more formal agreement than the ADM and requires the involvement of a medical doctor and another health professional. At this level, the appointed CDM must: (i) explain all relevant information and options to the person, (ii) assist the person to obtain this information if needed, (iii) find out their will and preference and (iv) assist that person to communicate this. The CDM must also discuss with the person

---

4   Reasons put forward for the delay in implementing the Act include the time required to establish both the new decision support service of the Mental Health Commission and the codes of practice for health and social care professionals.

known alternatives and likely outcomes of the decision and must attempt to ensure that the decision is implemented as far as possible. At the time of appointing a CDM, the person must be able to understand the nature and consequences of their decision in the context of the available choices (Donnelly, 2019).

At the highest level of decision-making, the court may make a declaration of incapacity regarding a specific matter or matters and may appoint a decision-making representative (DMR) to act as a substitute decision-maker for the person. This type of decision-making, replaces the former Ward of Court legislation (Regulation Lunacy Act, 1871). Again, in keeping with the principle of presumed capacity, substitute decision-making may only ever be used as a last resort when the court has found that the decision-making-support framework cannot be used.

The ADMCA also makes provision under health care directives to enable a person to appoint a designated health care representative (HCR) to make decisions on their behalf about their physical or mental health care. These decisions will be null and void if the person is admitted involuntarily to hospital under mental health legislation. The ADMCA also makes provision for the person to appoint an EPA to cover all kinds of decision-making in relation to personal welfare or property and affairs (Flynn, 2018).

Like with other levels of supportive decision-making, when appointing an HCR or EPA the person must demonstrate that they have mental capacity. Important too is the fact that under the ADMCA, decisions are not made on the basis of best interests. Rather all decision-makers and supports must act in accordance with a set of principles that: (i) encourage the participation of the person, (ii) take cognizance of the person's past and present will and preference, (iii) take into account the person's beliefs and values and (iv) other factors the person would be likely to consider had they that ability (Donnelly, 2019).

In Ireland, despite the passing of this visionary legislation, prolonged delays in its implementation mean that substitute models of decision-making as opposed to supportive models, continue to be used and many family caregivers continue to behave in a paternalistic way and see themselves as proxy or surrogate decision-makers (Donnelly et al., 2018). There is also evidence of a reluctance on the part of Irish people including those who develop dementia in later life to engage in care planning in their earlier years (Tan et al., 2019) and a reluctance on the part of older adults today to plan for the future. A red sea poll, recently revealed that 80% of Irish adults have not thought or talked about where they would wish to be cared for should they become seriously ill and just 5% have documented their preferred place of care:<//www.safeguardingireland.org/80-have-not-considered-where-they-would-like-to-be-cared-for>.

Decision-making, autonomy and the person with dementia

There are different stages in the course of dementia where the individual's decision-making rights may be compromised and their personhood and autonomy undermined. The first is at the very early stages when a delayed diagnosis and its non-disclosure can undermine autonomy rights (ADI, 2011) and threaten personhood. At the early stages, a person can usually still engage in important decision-making about issues relevant to their lives (Milne, 2010; Brooker and Latham, 2016). Examples here include, making or updating a will and engaging in advanced care planning such as appointing an HCR or an EPA. Protections like these can only be legally drawn up when a person still has mental capacity (Flynn, 2018). This is why an early/timely diagnosis (see Chapter 3) and its ethical disclosure is critically important, as it can promote personhood and dignity, maximize autonomy (ADI, 2011) and empower that person to take ownership of their illness (Gilliard et al., 2005). Conversely, the absence of a timely diagnosis and its disclosure can seriously compromise the autonomy rights of the individual.

In Ireland the NDS explicitly states that people living with dementia should be: 'facilitated and supported to live and die well in their chosen environment including their own home or nursing home, if that is their choice' (p. 25). This right to autonomy and choice is also reiterated in the global action plan on the public health response to dementia (WHO,

2017). Yet in Ireland the absence of government commitment to delivering adequate home care services acts as a barrier to enabling the person with dementia exercise their right to live at home in the community. One Irish study has shown that in around 50% of cases, the admission of older people including those with dementia to nursing homes could have been avoided if appropriate home care services were available (Donnelly et al., 2016). This paucity of adequate home care services including IHCP for people with dementia along with the lack of choice in models of long-term residential care (O'Shea et al., 2019) also serves to undermine peoples' rights to autonomy.

Often at transition times, as for example, the transition from acute care to long-term residential care, decisions that will have far-reaching consequences on the daily life of the individual are rushed into and made *for the person* rather than *with the person*. These decisions are often made in busy and noisy environments, problematic for decision-making and sometimes in the absence of any attempt made to engage with the person for whom the decision matters most. It is not unusual that at these transition times, the person's cognitive impairment will be severe and their memory, comprehension and verbal skills will be deficient. For this reason, family members may refrain from informing their relative about the impending move, believing that the information communicated will neither be understood nor retained. A small-scale qualitative study conducted in Ireland some years back, showed that families often chose not to inform their relative about the planned relocation to a nursing home or misrepresented information about the transfer (Bobersky, 2013).

Whilst there is no easy way to negotiate these transitions, deceiving a person or choosing to withhold information simply because the person lacks capacity is unethical. Also, in the context of decision-making, the emphasis on mental capacity may not be most important. What may be more important, is choosing the right time to communicate with the individual, remembering that participation in decision-making can vary from full participation, to more collaborative decision-making (O'Connor and Purves, 2009) to at the very least, being informed and communicated with in a supportive, non-threatening way. What may also be important is providing comfort from anxiety, promoting personhood and acknowledging the individual's emotional response (Tilse et al., 2009).

Finally, much has been written about the autonomy rights of older people resident in long-stay care (see, e.g., McCormack, 2004; Boyle, 2008; Murphy and Welford, 2012; ADI, 2013; Alzheimer Europe, 2017; O'Shea et al., 2019) and how because of dementia these rights may be compromised. Loss of autonomy in long-stay residential care can occur for a number of reasons. These include, poor staff-resident ratios, the absence of staff training, poorly designed environments, rigid nursing home policies that fail to offer choice and place an undue emphasis on safety and protection (Beard, 2004) and the inappropriate use of surveillance and/or assistive technologies. This issue of the ethical use of technologies in long-stay residential care is most important in relation to personhood and autonomy rights (Astell, 2006). There is nothing inherently wrong with the use of such technologies provided they are introduced for the right reason, namely to preserve personhood (Kitwood, 1997a), promote autonomy, reduce risk (Robinson et al., 2007) and ultimately benefit the individual. However, if technologies are used to restrict freedom without the person's consent, then such practices are unethical and breach the individual's human rights (Welsh et al., 2003).

Conclusions

This chapter has returned the spotlight to the individual living with dementia and to important concepts including personhood, capacity, autonomy and decision-making. In the introductory section it was argued that representations of personhood and autonomy have changed significantly over time as has our understanding of dementia. It was suggested that dementia is not just a condition of the mind, the brain and memory but it is also a syndrome that impacts on selfhood, and on a person's positioning in a world that places inordinate value on rational thinking and mental capacity. We need to move beyond homing in exclusively on the pathology of dementia and see the person in a more contextualized dynamic way, conscious that all our interactions with that person will greatly impact on their subjective experiences.

A central theme underpinning this chapter is the important role we all play helping to preserve the individual's personhood, their right to autonomy and to participate as far as possible in important decisions affecting their lives. Valuing people who have dementia, irrespective of the severity of their cognitive impairment, protecting their autonomy and promoting personhood should be a key ethical principle guiding all policy and practice. The final part of the chapter provides an overview of the Irish ADMCA highlighting the fact that when fully enacted, this legislation will help to protect the autonomy rights of people living with dementia. The chapter concludes by exploring some critical stages in the course of dementia where the individual's decision-making abilities may be compromised and their personhood and autonomy placed at risk.

CHAPTER 7

Residential care

> Residential care does not reside in the building or its facilities but rather in the spirit of the people within.
>
> (Alan Gilsenan, 2010)

Introduction

In this chapter attention turns to the person, who at some stage in the course of the illness may have to leave home and enter long-term residential care. What type of long-term care facilities are available in Ireland to support that person's complex needs? Do people have a choice regarding their preferred care option and who pays for their long-term care? What proportion of people in long-term residential care in Ireland have dementia and what factors determine their admission? Why might the built and psychosocial environment in long-term residential care be important for a person with dementia? How does Ireland compare with other European countries whose history of population ageing and of designing dementia services is more advanced? These along with other questions will be answered in this chapter. But first attention is turned to a brief overview of the main features of Irish long-term care policy and to some of the most significant changes that have occurred in that policy landscape over the last fifteen years.

Irish long-term care policy

The key service providers

In Ireland, long-term residential care for older people is provided through the public, voluntary and private sectors. The private sector, by far the largest provider, accounts for about three quarters of all beds and here long-term care is delivered in private nursing homes (Daly, 2018). The public sector accounts for about one fifth of all provision and here long-term care is delivered through HSE extended care and welfare homes. The voluntary sector accounts for the remainder: here long-term care is delivered in voluntary homes, welfare homes or hospitals and provided by charity and religious groups (Daly, 2018). Regardless of the sector, most providers of long-term care beds in Ireland are funded by the state and most long-term care facilities are nursing homes (O'Shea et al., 2019).

Despite government policy that repeatedly purports to support community care policy over residential care policy for older people (Robins, 1988; O'Shea and O'Reilly, 1999; DOHC, 1994, 2001), in Ireland, an inbuilt policy bias exists favouring residential care. This is reflected in the fact that Irish people have an entitlement to long-term residential care but no similar entitlement to home care services. Furthermore the Exchequer spends almost three times as much on residential care compared with home care. For example, in 2017, the budget allocated for the Nursing Home Support Scheme (NHSS) was €940 million (Daly, 2018) but for the same year, spending on home-based care (home help and home care packages) was estimated to be €367 million (Department of Public Expenditure and Reform, 2018). Despite this lack of entitlement to home care services, there have been other important changes in Ireland affecting older peoples' entitlement to and experience of long-term residential care services and the section to follow will now address these.

Legislative and policy changes

The Irish residential care landscape has undergone significant change over more than a decade. A catalyst for this change was probably the

Leas Cross exposé that occurred in Ireland in 2005, when undercover reporters went into a private nursing home in Dublin and highlighted the type of neglect and systematic abuse that was taking place there (Prime Time, 2005). Soon after, a government commissioned inquiry led to the publication of an expert report based on the review of medical records (O'Neill, 2006). A year later, (2007), a new Health Act was passed and the Health Information Quality Authority (HIQA) was established.

The Health Act (2007) and the establishment of HIQA heralded the beginning of significant reform in how long-term residential care settings for older people in Ireland would operate in terms of registration and inspection. Prior to this, only nursing homes operated by private and voluntary providers were inspected by the HSE and the public sector was exempt. However, the new Health Act (2007) required that all designated centres whether run by the HSE, by private providers or by voluntary organizations, must be registered and inspected. The passing of the Health Act (2007) meant that all future nursing home registration would be dependent on providers delivering safe, high quality care in suitable surroundings. All nursing homes would have to register with HIQA and undergo regular inspections in compliance with national residential care standards (HIQA, 2009).

For the older person in need of nursing home care, the Nursing Home Support Scheme Act (NHSS, 2009), popularly known as the Fair Deal Scheme and administered through the HSE, introduced some equity in a previously discriminatory system. It replaced the previous system of out-of-pocket pension-based payments for some public long-term care and co-payments through government subventions for private care (Daly, 2018); a system underpinned by the Health (Nursing Home) Act (1990) and the Code of Practice for Nursing Homes (1995).

The rationale underpinning the NHSS (2009) was to make residential care more accessible, affordable, by removing inequities and improving the state's role in delivering and meeting costs (<ntpf.ie/home/nhss.htm>). A gatekeeping system was introduced whereby only older people assessed as in need of long-term care would qualify for state funding. Under this scheme, the person's contribution towards the cost of care is based on an assessment of their income and assets[1]. If the person is part of a couple, this assessment is based on half of the couple's combined income and assets. Broadly speaking the person makes a contribution of 80% of their assessable income and 7.5% of the value of any assets. However, the first €36,000 of a person's assets (or double that amount i.e. €72,000 if that person is part of a couple) is disregarded. Regarding this financial assessment, a person's principal place of residence is only included for assessment at 7.5% during the first three years that person is in long-term care. Thereafter, this component of payment is exempt. However, the 7.5% payment on all other assets is on-going for as long as that person remains in long-term residential care. Although this new system works reasonably well, the Exchequer continues to fund about three-quarters of the cost of long-term care (Daly, 2018) and given population ageing there are growing concerns that the system will no longer be sustainable. Already it is noted that demand for long-term care beds in Ireland outstrips supply (Cushman and Wakefield, 2017).

Interestingly, for the provider, inequities continue to exist with the NHSS (the mechanism through which the cost of long-term care for most nursing home residents is funded). Private and voluntary providers receive significantly smaller payments for care per resident from the HSE compared with public providers (Shanahan, 2019). Whilst the HSE administers the scheme and facilitates payments to individual nursing homes, the National Treatment and Purchase Fund (NTPF) establishes the prices payable to approved private and voluntary nursing home providers, but plays no role in establishing costs paid to the public sector. These costs are set down internally by the HSE.

At the end of 2019, the agreed average weekly price paid to private and voluntary nursing home operators was €974, whilst the price per resident paid to public nursing home operators (HSE nursing homes) under the NHSS was €1615 (Shanahan, 2019). Furthermore, a range of therapies, specialist treatments, recreational activities and other miscellaneous items included at no extra cost in HSE nursing homes are excluded for payment under the cost component of the NHSS in private and voluntary nursing

---

1   For a more detailed overview of the cost component of this scheme see https://www2.hse.ie/services/fair-deal-scheme/about-the-fair-deal-scheme.html

homes. This has been the subject of heated debate over the years without resolution and will be returned to later in this chapter.

Facts about people with dementia living in long-term residential care

Proportion of beds occupied by people with dementia

Estimates have recently been generated on the number of older people living in nursing homes in Ireland (Pierse et al., 2019). Based on a bed occupancy rate of 96% (HIQA, 2016), there were 27,125 men and women living in long-stay residential care in Ireland in 2016. Also based on nursing home dementia prevalence rates found in the UK CFAS11 study (Matthews et al., 2016), it was estimated that about 19,530 of these Irish people (72% of all residents) had dementia.. These figures concur with earlier estimates where it was found that 89% of nursing home residents had a cognitive impairment of whom 69% probably had dementia (Cahill et al., 2010). Like in the UK (Prince et al., 2014), in Ireland, therefore the care of people who have dementia is the main focus of long-term residential care in Ireland (Cahill et al., 2010).These older people with dementia who live in nursing homes are generally very frail. Most will have high levels of functional impairment with about 40% being either bed-bound or chair-bound (Pierse et al., 2019).

Gaps in knowledge base

There are still gaps in our knowledge about the care of people with dementia in residential care settings in Ireland (Cahill et al., 2010; Pierse et al., 2019). We do not know the main reasons why some people must leave home and enter residential care, as to date no longitudinal study has been conducted on this topic. We suspect that reasons for nursing home admission are not that dissimilar from those cited in the international literature. These include: (i) factors associated with the primary caregiver, such as caregiver burden (Horttana et al., 2007; Etters et al., 2008; Luppa et al., 2010) and ill-health (Park et al., 2004; Schulz et al., 2004); (ii) factors associated with the person with dementia, such as severity of the condition and old age (Cepoiu-Martin et al., 2016), functional and cognitive decline and the presence of *behaviours that challenge* (Gaugler et al., 2007; Cepoiu-Martin et al., 2016) and (iii) factors associated with the care system, such as absence or inadequacy of informal support (Caron et al., 2006; Sussman and Regehr, 2009).

Qualitative research in Ireland (Argyle et al., 2010) showed that a myriad of inter-related factors determined the admission of people with dementia into nursing home care. Although small-scale, that study identified caregiver burden, lack of formal and informal support, a decline in health, the demands of caregiving and role conflict as determinants. Another qualitative study (Bobersky, 2013) that looked at reasons for admission to specialist care units of people diagnosed with dementia, revealed additional factors including safety concerns, *behaviours that challenge* and poorly adapted housing as precipitants. A more recent Irish study referred to earlier (see Chapter 5) based on a sample of spouse caregivers has shown that factors associated with the individual (such as psychosis and severe functional impairment) and factors associated with the caregiver (such as age and gender) increased the likelihood of people with dementia being admitted to nursing homes (Walsh et al., 2019).

Across most EU Member States there is widespread support for the concept of *ageing in place* policies (Eurobarometer, 2007), a term used to describe a person living in a place of their choice as they age and for as long as they wish. *Ageing in place* is also very salient for people who have dementia for whom familiarity and connectivity are so important (O'Shea et al., 2019). Yet we have no data in Ireland on pathways through dementia care, including the multiple moves a person may make prior to their admission to long-stay residential care and subsequently. Nor do we know the extent to which home adaptation grants or assistive technologies may have prevented these people from being admitted to nursing homes. We also do not know the average length of time people with dementia spend in nursing homes. Overseas research shows that this is longer for a person with dementia compared to other residents (A&N, 2011). Nor do we know what proportion of people living in Irish nursing homes, develop dementia after their admission and what type of diagnostic and post-diagnostic services do they receive. There is also an absence of information on the location of death of people with dementia, as for example, what proportion of residents move from nursing homes into hospitals or hospices at end of life and what proportion are offered palliative care services either within nursing homes or outside. An Irish study on end of life and dementia conducted several years ago showed that dementia was very seldom recorded on death certificates as a cause of death even though *death due to dementia* was an inclusion criterion for this same study (Cahill et al., 2012). These are all areas fruitful for future research.

The continuum of care for people living with dementia in the USA and Europe

As witnessed in other health care sectors, such as mental health and care for people with an intellectual disability, a gradual recalibration of care models for frail older people with dementia has emerged across Europe in the last three decades (Verbeek et al., 2009; De Lange et al., 2011; Verbeek, 2011; Cadigan et al., 2012; Ausserhofer et al., 2016). The recalibration is reflected in a shift from institutional care to more small-scale psychosocial and person-centred models of care (Verbeek, 2011, O'Shea et al., 2019). In the USA the so-called *humanization* of long-term care settings commenced as early as the 1970's with the pioneering work of the late Powel Lawton. Lawton, a clinical psychologist, was probably the first to identify the close association between the physical environment and older peoples' quality of life (Eisdorfer and Lawton, 1973) and to argue that as a person's ability declines, environmental support becomes increasingly more important. He argued that all too often, older people adapt their behaviour to fit their environment rather than having the environment be adapted to accommodate that behaviour. His many works (see, e.g., Lawton et al., 1996, 1997, 1999 and Lawton, 2001) have made a very significant contribution to dementia care. Lawton's work preceded policy reconfigurations such as the Eden Alternative, Green Houses and other new models of nursing homes that have more recently placed an emphasis on activities involving fresh air, plants and domestic animals (McLean, 2010).

Across Europe, this recalibration in care settings was first witnessed in Scandinavian countries. For example, in 1987, Denmark passed new legislation whereby all institutional care for older people was suspended and in Sweden, residential care was replaced with special housing in various forms in 1992 (Daatland et al., 2015). Since the 1990s the Netherlands has also trail blazed in the area of providing frail older people including those with dementia, with a suite of different accommodation options (Pot and de Lange, 2010; De Lange, 2011). The Danish, Swedish and Dutch models are organized on a social rather than medical model of care (Malmberg and Zarit, 1993; Verbeek, 2011). These models emphasize the maintenance of personal autonomy and competencies through a combination of environmental features, meaningful activities and facilitative relationships developed between staff and residents.

The models are underpinned by values such as individualization, personhood, choice, identity and connectivity (Verbeek, 2011; O'Shea et al., 2019). Models like these have emerged as it is argued that traditional large-scale nursing homes with a strongly medical and nursing based approach, provide little guidance for care (Kahn, 1975; Taft et al., 1997; Verbeek et al., 2009) and that a domestic environment can promote good quality of life (AE, 2017). Innovative models of long-term care that promote quality of life including respect for privacy have been endorsed by organizations such as WHO, the International Association of Gerontology and Geriatrics and the Institute of Medicine in the USA (Ausserhofer et al., 2016) along with the OECD (2015).

The continuum of care for people living with dementia in Ireland

Despite calls for alternatives to the conventional nursing home model (O'Shea and O'Reilly, 1999), innovation in the design of long-term care facilities has been very slow to develop in Ireland and there are few alternatives to the traditional nursing home model available to people who have dementia (Cahill et al., 2012; Bobersky, 2013; Convery, 2014; Cahill et al., 2015a). A recent and welcome breakthrough has been the call by the HSE for a review of a range of long-term care options for people living with dementia. This review on the continuum of care (O'Shea et al., 2019) has uncovered only one dementia village situated in rural Ireland. The same review identified few housing-with-care models equipped to meet the complex needs of people living with dementia. Sheltered housing was also found to be limited in Ireland with little information available on the extent to which this model currently supports the sometimes complex accommodation needs of people living with dementia.

There are also few specialist care units in Ireland, either stand-alone or attached to more traditional nursing homes for people diagnosed with dementia. A large national survey of Irish nursing homes undertaken by the DSIDC, some years ago revealed that only 11% operated specialist care units (Cahill et al., 2015a). The survey of over 600 nursing homes found that the private sector provided the main bulk of dementia care (63%) but compared with the public sector received significantly less funding. Nationally, there were significant inequities in the location and numbers of specialist units available to older people. Even when units were identified, their size did not always comply with international norms (Cahill et al., 2015a).

There is also a history in Ireland of new often large-scale nursing homes being built sometimes in remote areas on the outskirts of cities (Hourihan, 2018) or on the borders of villages or townships where residents are sometimes socially marooned, separated from their local communities and from people, places, activities and surroundings once familiar to them. This is probably because land is cheaper in such areas; developers may not always prioritize issues relating to optimal dementia care and civic society tends to place little pressure on governments for creative thinking and policy reform.

Models of care in other European countries

In Scandinavian countries like Norway and Sweden, assisted-living dwellings or small-scale group-living facilities for persons with dementia are a common feature of the aged care landscape. These facilities are often highly visible in the community, accessible by public transport and located in the heart of neighbourhoods, next to parks, cinemas, galleries, schools, playgrounds, shopping centres and so on. Familiarity, connectivity and consistency are so important for people living with dementia (Aminzadeh et al., 2010) and care facilities located near where the person with dementia once lived and serviced by the same care staff that once offered that person in-home supports, will promote social engagement and enhance a person's ability to remain connected into a familiar neighbourhood and community.

It is unclear why alternate models of long-term care have not been developed in Ireland. One reason may be that for service planning and development, policy makers need empirical data. They need valid and reliable information on costs and outcomes to make wise decisions on resource allocation (O'Shea et al., 2019) but the evidence on the cost-benefit effectiveness of these more innovative approaches has not been that compelling (de Rooij et al., 2011) with some studies providing contradictory findings (Wimo, 1991; Verbeek, 2013). A difficulty in Ireland too is that from a service perspective health and housing are not seen as unified or interconnected concepts. There have also been failures of co-ordination and integration in Ireland with silos developing that have led to the separation of care, housing, environment and transport for people with dementia. The dominance of the biomedical model (see Chapter 2) in policy-making could also make it difficult to think in a more holistic way about care provision.

People with dementia who live in nursing homes often feel disconnected from their local community, lonely and may crave familiar people, hobbies and activities (Cahill and Diaz-Ponce, 2011). With the right support in the right place at the right time, even residents with a moderately severe dementia, can continue to access local networks and conveniences familiar to them, such as shops, parks, hairdressers, pubs, cinemas, church, town hall and so on. In designated dementia inclusive communities this model of long-term care is likely to work very well. However, in Ireland a major disconnect exists between housing and health care services; between social care needs and health care needs; between budget allocation for older people's home care services and nursing home services and between community and residential care. In some European countries these boundaries are becoming more fluid (Glendinning, 2018), while in Ireland they remain rigid and often impenetrable.

Despite a burgeoning body of research conducted in the area, it is also difficult to tease out variables that contribute to quality of life in long-term residential care in the absence of large-scale crossover studies. For example, although there is evidence that small-scale living can be beneficial for people who have dementia, the 'Living Arrangements for People with Dementia study in the Netherlands' (Willemse et al., 2011) showed that small-scale living could be achieved even more successfully in traditional nursing homes (compared with group-living facilities) when living areas were broken up into smaller spaces (Pot, 2013). Other research challenges here include selecting large sample sizes, conducting longitudinal research where attrition rates may be high, choosing the right outcome measures and the right unit of analysis. Certainly, the evidence that *is compelling* is that older Irish people including those who have dementia want to remain in their own homes (Keogh et al., 2019; O'Shea et al., 2019; Rochford-Brennan, 2019).

The built and psychosocial environment

Accordingly, the goal of any long-term residential care facility should be to make the environment small-scale familiar and distinct from any institutional setting, essentially creating a home away from home. As far as possible, residents should be surrounded with their personal belongings and memorabilia that tell their story, helping to keep them connected to their families, friends and community and to what matters most to them, including links to earlier stages of their lives. Feeling at home is so important for the person diagnosed with dementia who is likely to be facing increasing dependencies, disruptions and disconnections (Aminzadeh et al., 2010). The common meanings and functions of home such as constancy, affinity, belongingness, identity and familiarity should inform the design ethos and organization of care in all long-stay care facilities.

Good environmental design is said to be as vital to the resident's care as is staffing and the ethos of care (Calkins, 1988). The physical environment should be used as a therapeutic tool and every aspect of it manipulated to promote personhood, dignity and well-being and to maximize independence and minimize risk. A bedroom that resonates with the resident's identity, embraces familiarity, connectivity and a sense of belonging will probably help that person to better deal with transitions. Bedrooms should be personalized with the resident's own furniture, photographs and mementos in evidence to reinforce identity and promote well-being. A homely nursing home with no slavish commitment to communal care will also facilitate psychological adjustment (Stokes, 2011).

In this context, it is important to emphasize that most Irish nursing homes strive to create supportive personalized environments that are domestic-like and promote a good quality of life. Many Irish nursing homes are highly successful at achieving this: they subscribe to this *new culture of care* and have creative programmes on offer, catering for their residents' diverse needs including their need to take exercise both indoors and outdoors. However, others struggle because the built environment is not customized for people who have dementia and this makes it very difficult for front-line staff to deliver personalized care in a dignity-enhancing way.

The design and lay-out of internal rooms should communicate to the individual the function of that room. Safe and secure surroundings complete with cueing and signage will make it easier for residents to remain independent, exercise autonomy and move about unassisted. Easy access to a carefully designed multisensory outdoor area is a human right (Cahill, 2018a) and every resident should have access to fresh air for exercise and contact with nature (Argyle et al., 2016). Indeed, any interface with the outdoor environment will assist with sleep and wake patterns (Brawley, 2001) and with seasonal orientation (Gilliard and Marshall, 2012). A policy whereby residents have the freedom to go outdoors and access fresh air should be written into the philosophy of every long-term care environment (Welsh et al., 2003) and implemented.

However, feeling at home requires more than customizing the built environment. It also depends on the psychosocial environment; the care process and on the range and quality of relationships including friendships that develop within. Staff, resident and family interactions are all intrinsic to the care process. Families can sometimes feel sidelined by busy front-line staff who are often under huge pressure with multiple demands on their time. Yet families are integral to the functioning of long-term care facilities as they can provide a rich source of support helping staff understand the best way to interact with their relative (Fossey, 2010).

Caring for a person with dementia can be extremely stressful, especially for care staff who are at the front line. Nursing home staff, most of whom are women and whose responsibilities are enormous, generally work long hours and are not well paid. For every one resident in their care, front-line staff will have at least two sets of clients, the resident and that person's family members. These family members may not always be in agreement with each other or indeed with care staff about how care plans are devised and how formal care is delivered. This places further tension and strain on busy nursing home care staff.

Many nursing home staff get to know their residents so well and so personally and care for them as they would care for their own close family members. They know what makes the resident happy, sad, angry, anxious, agitated and so on. They can often anticipate their every need and difficulty. For many staff employed in nursing homes, caregiving is a lot more than work and the injunction to care experienced can extend way beyond the call of duty. Caring for, caring about and being bonded to residents, means that when a resident dies, many staff also experience significant loss and grief. This may be at a time when they are under huge pressure to admit a new resident, help that person adjust to the new environment and deal with the anxieties of the new resident's close family members. Nursing home staff must be supported for the hard physical and emotional work they undertake delivering dementia care. They must be given time out to debrief following critical incidents. They must be encouraged and facilitated to undertake regular training. Most importantly, they must be valued and better paid for the very stressful work they undertake. If staff are not valued and nurtured, it is unlikely they will be able to deliver personalized quality care. Good leadership, careful mentoring and ongoing staff training and support are so important for quality of care.

Irrespective of how well a nursing home environment is designed, if the ethos of care is rigid and if no choice and sense of homeliness are promoted, the resident's quality of life may be seriously affected. In nursing homes where an over-reliance continues to be placed on clinical technical care, this must be replaced with a focus on person-centred, personalized care, taking due cognizance of the individual's life story and biography. Recreational activities known to improve quality of life such as reminiscence programmes (O'Shea et al., 2014) and activities that provide psychosocial stimulation such as music therapy (Fang et al., 2017), CST (Clare and Woods, 2004) and creative therapies such as: art, pottery, aromatherapy need to be promoted and funded in residential care settings. Domestic activities such as watering plants, sorting, baking, sewing or sensory interventions such tactile stimulation are also equally important for resident well-being.

A key difficulty for private and voluntary providers in Ireland is that therapies and recreational activities are not included under the cost components of the NHSS (2009). This means that payments for therapies and for activity programmes must be recouped as additional out-of-pocket expenses. Ironically the cost of drug treatments such as antipsychotic medication sometimes prescribed by medical doctors attending nursing home residents who have dementia, is generally reimbursed by the government. This is because most older people will have medical cards. However, there is no equivalent reimbursement scheme to pay for employing a physiotherapist, psychologist, social worker, occupational therapist, speech and language therapist and so on. Nor is funding available to pay for an activity coordinator for recreational activities like reminiscence, life story work, CST, pottery, art, pet therapy, aromatherapy and so on. The current policy bias that favours medical prescribing over social prescribing needs to be challenged. The value of non-pharmacological interventions must be acknowledged and nursing homes must be appropriately reimbursed for their use.

Conclusions

Nursing home care is the predominant model of long-term residential care available to older people who have dementia in Ireland and this chapter has outlined the type of reform that has taken place in Irish nursing homes over the last fifteen years. It has addressed the question of who in Ireland are the main providers of these nursing homes; what proportion of people in nursing homes are likely to have dementia and what is their level of disability? It has argued that while the drive to improve quality of life for older people living in nursing homes has been a welcome feature of Irish aged care reform, no similar drive exists to design and trial more innovative models of long-term care. This is at a time when alternative models to nursing homes such as small-scale assisted-living facilities, housing-with-care, sheltered housing and dementia villages have gained popularity across Europe and globally. The chapter has shown that most people in Ireland who have dementia and need long-term residential care, live in traditional large-scale nursing homes, many of which are not purpose-built or designed to meet their unique and complex needs. For front-line care staff, large-scale congregate nursing home environments that are not customized for a person with dementia will make dementia care very stressful.

Irish people have a legal entitlement to nursing home care and to state financial support for this care following assessment, but they have no similar legal entitlement to remain at home with appropriate home care services. This policy bias now needs to be challenged. There is a need for a shift in the balance of care, away from nursing home models and towards alternate potentially more cost-effective models of home-based long-term care. We need to listen carefully to the preferences of older Irish people including those with dementia who wish to remain in their own homes. A greater emphasis needs to be placed on home adaptation, universal design and technological solutions to help the person remain safe in their own home, surrounded by what is familiar to them. In the event that this is no longer possible, we need to provide a suite of long-term care options including housing-with-care, group-living facilities, sheltered housing, and specialist care units that will resemble a home away from home.

We are now at a critical juncture regarding the future direction of long-term residential care for people with dementia in Ireland. Population ageing, along with an expected increase in dementia prevalence rates and an expected decline in the availability of informal caregivers will place very significant demands on fiscal resources. Like other Western countries, the country now needs to confront the question of the sustainability of long-term care funding systems. Will the government's planned statutory home care scheme (soon to be introduced) reduce future demand for long-term nursing home beds? Will the government act on findings emerging from the recent continuum of care report on dementia care services and introduce a broader range of long-term care options? Will the country witness a reversal in spending on older peoples' services with a funding shift from residential care to home-based services? Who knows the answers to these questions, only time will tell. However, what is certain is that planning for the future is now more urgent that ever before and any substantive change will require political will, supportive policies and legislative reform.

CHAPTER 8

Conclusions

As I write this final chapter, I am conscious that we are in the middle of a world pandemic of a magnitude never witnessed before, well certainly not in my lifetime. To date Covid-19 has taken its toll on many thousands of human lives around the world, especially in countries like China, Iran, Italy, Spain, France, the UK and more recently the USA and Brazil. Many of those most severely affected by the virus are older people and front-line health and social care staff. Amongst older people, a sizeable proportion are frail men and women living in nursing homes, many of whom have dementia and are unable to communicate their fears, needs, desires, loneliness and possible sense of abandonment. During a pandemic crisis of this magnitude, older people with dementia are extremely vulnerable: many will not have had the opportunity to see their spouses, children and other loved ones for long periods, nor understand the gravity of the pandemic and the need for social distancing and self-isolation. The human impact of this pandemic is huge and its economic and social impact will also be very profound. Therefore, I am writing this chapter conscious that we are approaching extremely challenging times where resources will be more scarce than ever before.

As several of the chapters in this book have shown, much has happened in Ireland over the last decade on the ageing and dementia front. Significant advances have occurred in policy, research and practice. As shown in Chapter 1, many of these advances were spearheaded by the Atlantic Philanthropies' investment programme in dementia in Ireland, that first commenced in 2005. Other advances have occurred since 2014, when Ireland's first NDS was launched. The NDS was a policy plan that was different as it came with a budget and it had buy-in from all of the key stakeholders. Consequently the NDS had political ownership. These were all factors crucial to its successful implementation.

The NDS was different too as it was embedded in the principles of personhood and citizenship. These principles reflect a commitment to seeing the *person* rather than the *dementia* and to recognizing that no matter how severe the cognitive loss is, there is a core self that remains recognizable and fundamentally intact in every human being. An earlier action plan on dementia had been developed (O'Shea and O'Reilly, 1999) but that plan lacked resources; it had no veritable political ownership and was never implemented. For that reason, dementia got lost. It was squeezed between health and social care and between mental health and physical health. Getting lost meant that very little happened. So, in Ireland we were starting from a very low baseline in terms of dementia services.

Since the launch of the NDS and the establishment of the NDO, various work streams have been developed to advance prioritized actions. These include: de-stigmatizing dementia and enhancing public and professional awareness and understanding, workforce education including the training of GPs and primary care staff, and the delivery of IHCP. More recently an ambitious programme of work to develop *dementia diagnostic and post-diagnostic pathways* is now underway and several research studies underpinning these programmes have been completed. Much of this recent work has been funded through government dormant accounts.

One important programme of low impact but high quality has been the introduction of post-diagnostic services to a small group of community-dwelling people who have dementia (see Chapter 3). Apart from offering more individualized supports, this programme has trained and mobilized health service professionals committed to best practice in dementia care and determined to make a difference. Work has also progressed in the acute care sector through the education of health care staff: the customization of some hospital environments to make them more dementia-friendly and a second audit of dementia in the acute care sector has taken place in Ireland. The ASI has also been at the fore in its advocacy work, service delivery, brain health, dementia inclusive community programmes and commissioned research. As a result of these along with many other dementia-related activities, considerable progress has been achieved within a relatively short period of time.

Aims of this book

My intention in writing this book was to try to document some of the core aspects of this *transformation process* that has helped to drive social and political change and improve the lives of some of the 55,000 people in Ireland estimated to have dementia. The intention was also to critically review and collate findings from Irish health service research on dementia, in order to provide a more contemporary overview of where Ireland currently stands, in relation to policy and practice development. The country is fortunate as there are engines of excellence located in certain parts of the island that continue to pump out new data, critical for future policy and service development. Their dedication to the area along with their in-depth painstaking work has made it easier for me to write several of these chapters.

In writing the book, it was not my intention to address unique situations and throughout the chapters, efforts have been made to keep the central message broad and to avoid providing information that might quickly get outdated. That message is that while dementia may strip people of their memory and cognitive abilities, it does not strip them of their humanity, dignity, right to autonomy and personhood. It is society and those of us deemed healthy and cognitively intact that do this through deficit-based policies, practices that can sometimes de-skill rather than empower and research that is not always inclusive of the individual's voice. By addressing each of these areas individually and collectively we can do a lot to support the person to function better and live well in a more inclusive world. Valuing the person and promoting their autonomy and dignity should be the main ethical concern for family caregivers and formal caregivers who must work together as partners or co-producers of care, recognizing each other's skills and expertise.

Limitations

Like in any book it is impossible to cover all topics comprehensively and I am conscious that more is happening in Ireland on the national dementia stage that has not been covered in these chapters. Examples here include the programme of research and training now underway at the Global Brain Health Institute at Trinity College Dublin: an ambitious project that has received very sizeable funding and involves the training of international fellows in dementia and brain health and the development of policy-related methods for dementia prevention. Other examples include the modelling work currently underway to develop a national dementia registry and led by researchers at Dublin City University. Yet another example is the establishment of the new assessment and diagnostic centre for people with intellectual disability and Alzheimer's disease led by staff in Trinity College Dublin. These initiatives along with others are at an early stage and the more long-term impact from these investments will not be known for some time. Now in drawing this book to a conclusion I want to return to another core theme underpinning virtually all of the earlier chapters. This theme relates to the complexities of dementia and of caregiving.

Concluding remarks

Complexities of dementia

Throughout the chapters I have tried to highlight the complexities that dementia poses for different groups of people. There are complexities for the individual, experiencing the symptoms, since these symptoms can be frightening, worrying, potentially embarrassing and are not always easily recognizable. The symptoms can be complicated by other health conditions and by delayed responses in poorly integrated health and social

Conclusions

care systems (see Chapters 3 and 4). There are complexities for GPs, attempting to provide their *patients* with a timely diagnosis in sometimes extremely challenging circumstances (see Chapter 3). There are complexities for other health care professionals and service providers, including busy front-line nursing home care staff, some of whom are working in facilities that are poorly customized for a condition like dementia; congregate environments that can make care delivery exceptionally challenging and stressful. There are also complexities for governments required to make decisions about the equitable allocation of resources when budgets are restricted and will probably be even more so in coming years. There are complexities for the public, fearful of dementia and trying to make sense of Alzheimer's disease given its changing definitions (see Chapter 1). Many of these complexities result in ethical and moral dilemmas that challenge our inner thoughts and cause us to reflect on our own personal frameworks, the meaning of life, our humanity and mortality.

Complexities of family caregiving

Throughout earlier chapters of this book, I have also highlighted the complexities confronting family caregivers supporting a loved one with dementia, of whom we know there are about 60,000 in Ireland. Often alone, many attempt to deliver personalized and dignity-enhancing care, while gauging the level of assistance that is acceptable to a close family member. Usually women, these informal caregivers are often wives or daughters who provide the main bulk of caring. Most want to care, but they also want to receive recognition from the government for the hard physical and emotional work they do behind closed doors. As shown in Chapter 5, many receive no financial support from the government for the services they deliver free of charge, nor do they receive much assistance from home care services or from other family members. Informal caregiving is both *labour* and *love*. However, the *love* component may quickly become eroded by the sheer enormity of the care tasks demanded and the *labour* component may also get overlooked by governments keen to emphasize the *caring about* rather than *caring for* aspects of informal care.

For many, caregiving also means having to balance a loved one's safety needs against their need for independence and autonomy and this can pose moral and ethical dilemmas. Understandably, family caregivers can become frustrated in a system that is poorly signposted, inadequately integrated and one that claims to favour home care over residential care yet provides no legal entitlement to relevant home care supports. Other complexities confronted by some include: juggling multiple care roles, combining paid work with family care and caring at a distance or essentially running two homes. Finally, there are complexities for many family caregivers attempting to respond to dementia-related *behaviours that challenge*, that can cause great distress and for which there are no immediate solutions. These behaviours can be potentially embarrassing, unpredictable, annoying and can cause sleep deprivation. They can result in tensions and arguments arising between the caregiver and the person being cared for because of that person's apparent 'insensitivities' to the emotional well-being of the family caregiver, usually the person who loves them most.

Future directions

We are now at an interesting juncture in Ireland in relation to dementia policy, research and practice. As shown throughout this book, much has happened to advance the national dementia agenda over a relatively short period of time. A new policy framework on dementia has been developed and since 2014 many of its key recommendations have been implemented. In 2015, the country passed new legislation on capacity and decision-making. This legislation when fully enacted will have significant ramifications for Irish people with dementia since it confers autonomy rights on the person whose mental capacity may be compromised. In this context it is regrettable that this important piece of legislation has not as yet been fully operationalized. Pressure now needs to be exerted on the government for its more widespread and immediate implementation.

Since 2018, Ireland has also ratified the UN Convention on the Rights of Persons with Disability (CRPD, 2006) which means that the government has entered into agreement at an international level to convert its principles into policy and practice. The country also has a very powerful self-advocacy movement through the Irish Working Group on Dementia that until recently has been chaired by Kathy Ryan and led by the ASI. At a European level, the Chairperson of the European Working Group is Dr Helen Rochford-Brennan, an inspirational Irish advocate and a person living with young-onset dementia.

Despite such progress, I am conscious that the original ring-fenced philanthropic funding allocated for dementia policy, practice and research has now run dry. Many of the new dementia services discussed in earlier chapters of this book and designed to improve quality of life have relied on dormant accounts and these accounts are unlikely to be sustainable in the future. This means that unless Exchequer funding for dementia becomes available, the *service transformation* process described in this book will very soon grind to a halt. The mid-term review of the implementation of the NDS highlighted the need for dedicated funding to be set aside for dementia service development (HSE, 2018). This funding needs to be realistic, taking cognizance of demographic projections and future estimates of incidence and prevalence rates of dementia.

There is also a need for a new focus to be placed on a small number of dementia-specific initiatives that have not been prioritized in the implementation of the NDS. One of these is the future training of Irish GPs in dementia diagnosis and disclosure. A key finding from the PREPARED project was that in order for an educational intervention to be effective, training should be delivered in small group format. GP training should be peer-facilitated and should take place in interactive workshops where the focus is on case-based clinical discussions. Since the completion of the PREPARED project, this type of peer-led dementia-specific interactive training, known to work well, is no longer available. These small GP-led interactive workshops focusing on dementia diagnosis, disclosure and management now need to be re-introduced and made available nationally.

There is also a need for standards of care to be developed for Irish memory clinics providing assessment and diagnostic services. Like in the

UK and in other countries, Irish memory clinics must be accredited and better integrated into the health care system with more visionary blended pathways developed between primary and secondary care services. Specialist out-reach support from memory clinic staff also needs to be made available to primary care managed dementia services. Memory clinics also need to be more proactive in offering the person diagnosed, better access to non-pharmacological interventions such as CR and CST. These types of services need to be embedded in the health and social care system.

Finally, at a national level, strong political leadership on the dementia stage is more vital than ever before and pressure must now be exerted on the government to develop a new national dementia strategy, since without a policy plan, there is every likelihood that dementia will once again get lost and forgotten. This new Irish dementia strategy must be embedded in the principles of human rights, personhood and citizenship; and flexible personalized home care services must constitute its central plank. The overarching goal must be for informal caregivers and formal caregivers to work together and provide the person diagnosed with dementia with the opportunity to live with dignity and enjoy a good quality of life. For how society views and treats its most vulnerable, reflects that society's fabric and character. We here in Ireland have within reach, the opportunity to make Ireland one of the best places in the world for people with dementia to grow old in, provided we start planning relevant services now.

References

A&N. (2011). *Position Statement No's 9 and 10 The Geriatricians' Perspective on Medical Services to Residential Aged Care Facilities (RCFs) in Australia.* Australian and New Zealand Society for Geriatric Medicine.

ADI. (2011). *The World Alzheimer Report 2011: The benefits of early diagnosis and intervention.* London: Alzheimer's Disease International, <https://www.alz.co.uk/ADI-conference-2011>, accessed 8 April 2020.

ADI. (2013). *The World Alzheimer Report 2013: An analysis of long-term care for dementia.* London: Alzheimer's Disease International. <https://www.alz.co.uk/research/world-report-2013>, accessed 8 April 2020.

ADI. (2015). *The World Alzheimer Report 2015, The Global Impact of Dementia: An analysis of prevalence, incidence, cost and trends.* London: Alzheimer's Disease International, <https://www.alz.co.uk/research/world-report-2015>, accessed 8 April 2020.

ADMCA. (2015). 'Assisted Decision-Making Capacity Act', <http://www.irishstatutebook.ie/eli/2015/act/64/enacted/en/html>, accessed 8 April 2020.

Aguirre, E., Spector, A., Streater, A., Hoe, J., Woods, B., and Orrell, M. (2012). 'Making a difference 2: An evidence-based group programme to offer maintenance cognitive stimulation therapy (CST) to people with dementia: The manual for group leaders', *Journal of Dementia Care.*

AE. (2012). *Annual Report 2012, The ethical issues linked to restrictions of freedom of people with dementia.* Luxembourg: Alzheimer Europe.

AE. (2014). *Dementia in Europe Yearbook. National care pathways for people with dementia living at home.* Luxembourg: Alzheimer Europe.

AE. (2016). *Discussion paper on ethical issues linked to the changing definitions/use of terms related to Alzheimer's disease.* Luxembourg: Alzheimer Europe.

AE. (2017). *Dementia in Europe Yearbook. Standards for residential care facilities in Europe.* Luxembourg: Alzheimer Europe.

AE. (2019). *Dementia in Europe Yearbook. Estimating the prevalence of dementia in Europe.* Luxembourg: Alzheimer Europe.

AS. (2011). 'Five pillar model of post diagnostic support', *Alzheimer Scotland*, <www.alzscot.org/five-pillars-model-of-post-diagnostic-support>, accessed 8 April 2020.

Alzheimer, A. (1907). 'Über eine eigenartige Erkrankung der Hirnrinde. Allgemeine Zeitschrift für Psychiatrie und Psychisch-Gerichtliche Medizin, 64'. In D. A.

Rottenberg and F. H. Hochberg (eds), *Neurological classics in modern translation*, 146–148. New York: Hafner Press.

Amieva, H., Robert, P. H., Grandoulier, A. S., Meillon, C., De Rotrou, J., Andrieu. S., Berr, C., Desgranges, B., Dubois, B., Girtanner, C., Joël, M. E., Lavallart, B., Nourhashemi, F., Pasquier, F., Rainfray, M., Touchon, J., Geneviève, C., and Dartigues J. F. (2016). 'Group and individual cognitive therapies in Alzheimer's disease: The ETNA3 randomized trial', *International Psychogeriatrics*, 28 (5), 707–717.

Aminzadeh, F., Dalziel, W. B., Molnar, F. J., and Garcia, L. J. (2010). 'Meanings, functions, and experiences of living at home for individuals with dementia at the critical point of relocation', *Journal of Gerontological Nursing*, 36 (6), 28–35.

Argyle, E., Dening, T., and Bartlett, P. (2016). 'Space, the final frontier: Outdoor access for people living with dementia', *Aging and Mental Health*, 21 (10), 1005–1006.

Argyle, E., Downs, M., and Tasker, J. (2010). 'Continuing to Care for People with Dementia: Irish family carers' experience of their relative's transition to a nursing home', <https://www.researchgate.net/publication/265574982_Continuing_to_Care_for_people_with_dementia_Irish_family_carers'_experience_of_their_relative's_transition_to_a_nursing_home>, accessed 8 April 2020.

ASI. (2019). *The Alzheimer Society of Ireland Submission to Political Parties on their General Election Manifestos*. Dublin: The Alzheimer Society of Ireland.

Astell, A. (2006). 'Technology and personhood in dementia care', *Quality in Ageing and Older Adults*, 7 (1), 15–25.

Ausserhofer, D., Deschodt, M., De Geest, S., van Achterberg, T., Meyer, G., Verbeek, H., Strømseng Sjetne, I., Malinowska-Lipień, I., Griffiths, P., Schlüter, W., Ellen, M., and Engberg, S. (2016). '"There's no place like home": A scoping review on the impact of homelike residential care models on resident-, family-, and staff-related outcomes', *Journal of the American Medical Directors Association*, 17 (8), 685–693.

Balasubramanian, A. B., Kawas, C. H., Peltz, C. B., Brookmeyer, R., and Corrada, M. M. (2012). 'Alzheimer disease pathology and longitudinal cognitive performance in the oldest-old with no dementia', *Neurology*, 79 (9), 915–921.

Banerjee, S. (2009). 'The use of antipsychotic medication for people with dementia: Time for action', A report for the Minister of State for Care Services, *Department of Health*, London, <https://www.jcpmh.info/wp-content/uploads/time-for-action.pdf>, accessed 8 April 2020.

Banerjee, S. (2015). 'A narrative review of evidence for the provision of memory services', *International psychogeriatrics*, 27 (10), 1583–1592.

Bartlett, R. (2000). 'Dementia as a disability: Can we learn from disability studies and theory?', *Journal of Dementia Care*, Sept/Oct, 33–36.

Bartlett, R. (2014). 'Citizenship in action: The lived experiences of citizens with dementia who campaign for social change', *Disability & Society*, 29(8), 1291–1304.

Bartlett, R., and O'Connor, D. (2007). 'From personhood to citizenship: Broadening the lens for dementia practice and research', *Journal of Ageing Studies*, 21, 107–118.

Bartlett, R., and O'Connor, D. (2010). *Broadening the dementia debate: Towards social citizenship*. Bristol: The Policy Press.

Beard, R. L. (2004). 'In their voices: Identity preservation and experiences of Alzheimer's disease', *Journal of Aging Studies*, 18 (4), 415–428.

Begley, E. (2009). *I know what it is but how bad does it get? Insights into the Lived Experience and Service Needs of People with Early-Stage Dementia* (unpublished PhD thesis), Trinity College Dublin.

Bello, V. M. E., and Schultz, R. R. (2011). 'Prevalence of treatable and reversible dementias: A study in a dementia outpatient clinic', *Dementia & neuropsychologia*, 5 (1), 44–47.

Benoit, M., Arbus, C., Blanchard, F., Camus, V., Cerase, V., Clement, J. P., Fremont, P., Guerin, O., Hazif-Thomas, C., Jeanblanc, F., Lafont, C., Moreaud, O., Pedra, M., Poncet, M., Richard Harston, S., Rigaud, A. S., Sotto Martin, M. E., Touchon, J., Vellas, B., Fitten,.L J., and Robert, P. H. (2006). 'Professional consensus on the treatment of agitation, aggressive behaviour, oppositional behaviour and psychotic disturbances in dementia', *The Journal of Nutrition, Health & Aging*, 10 (5), 410–415.

Bercholz, M., and FitzGerald, J. (2016). Recent trends in female labour force participation in Ireland. *Quarterly Economic Commentary*.49–81.

Berglund, E., Lytsy, P., and Westerling, R. (2015). Health and wellbeing in informal caregivers and non-caregivers: A comparative cross-sectional study of the Swedish general population', *Health and Quality of Life Outcomes*, 13 (1), 109.

Blackburn, S. (2005). *The Oxford dictionary of philosophy*. Oxford: OUP.

Blessed, G., Tomlinson, B. E., and Roth, M. (1968). 'The association between quantitative measures of dementia and of senile change in the cerebral grey matter of elderly subjects', *The British Journal of Psychiatry*, 114 (512), 797–811.

Bobersky, A. (2013). *It's been a good move. Transitions into care: Family caregivers', persons' with dementia, and formal staff members' experiences of specialist care unit placement* (unpublished PhD thesis), Trinity College Dublin, Ireland.

Bond, J. (2001). 'Sociological perspectives'. In C. Cantley (ed.), *A handbook of dementia care*, 44–61. Buckingham: Open University Press.

Bosco, A., Schneider, J., Coleston-Shields, D. M., Jawahar, K., Higgs, P., and Orrell, M. (2019). 'Agency in dementia care: Systematic review and meta-ethnography', *International Psychogeriatrics*, 31 (5), 627–642.

Boyle, G. (2008). 'Autonomy in long-term care: A need, a right or a luxury', *Disability and Society*, 23 (4), 299–310.

Bradshaw, A. (2020). 'Behind the headlines: Making sense of new aducanumab trial data', *Dementia in Society*. Alzheimer Europe, 29–31.

Braekhus, A., and Engedal, K. (2002). 'Diagnostic work-up of dementia – a survey among Norwegian general practitioners', *Brain Aging*, 2 (4), 63–67.

Brawley, E. (2001). 'Environmental design for Alzheimer's disease: A quality of life issue', *Aging and Mental Health*, 5 (S1), 79–83.

Brennan, S., Lawlor, B., Pertl, M. M., O'Sullivan, M., Begley, E., and O'Connell, C. (2017). *De-Stress: A study to assess health and well-being of spousal carers of people with dementia in Ireland*. Dublin: Alzheimer Society of Ireland.

Brock, D. W. (1988). 'Justice and the severely demented elderly', *Journal of Medicine and Philosophy*, 13 (1), 73–99.

Brodaty, H., and Donkin, M. (2009). 'Family caregivers of people with dementia', *Dialogues in Clinical Neuroscience*, 11 (2), 217.

Brooker, D., and Latham, I. (2016). *Person-centred dementia care: Making services better with the VIPS framework*. London: Jessica Kingsley.

Brooker, D., Fontaine, J. L., Evans, S., Bray, J., and Saad, K. (2014). 'Public health guidance to facilitate timely diagnosis of dementia: ALzheimer's Cooperative Valuation in Europe recommendations', *International Journal of Geriatric Psychiatry*, 29 (7), 682–693.

Buntinx, F., De Lepeleire, J., Paquay, L., Iliffe, S., and Schoenmakers, B. (2011). 'Diagnosing dementia: No easy job', *BMC Family Practice*, 12 (1), 60.

Byrne, E. J., Collins, D., and Burns, A. (eds) (2006). 'Behavioural and psychological symptoms of dementia-agitation'. In A. Burns and B. Winblad (eds), *Severe dementia*, 51–61. London: John Wiley & Sons.

Cadigan, R. O., Grabowski, D. C., Givens, J. L., and Mitchell, S. L. (2012). 'The quality of advanced dementia care in the nursing home: The role of special care units', *Medical Care*, 50 (10), 856.

Cahill, S. (1997). *I wish I could have hung on longer: Choices and dilemmas in dementia care* (PhD), University of Queensland.

Cahill, S. (1999). 'Caring in families: What motivates wives, daughters, and daughters-in-law to provide dementia care?', *Journal of Family Studies*, 5 (2), 235–247.

Cahill, S. (2018a). *Dementia and human rights*. Bristol: Policy Press.

References

Cahill, S. (2018b). 'Juggling Paid Work and Unpaid Care: Learning through cross-national comparisons'. *DG Employment, Social Affairs and Inclusion*, European Commission.

Cahill, S., and Diaz-Ponce, A. (2011). '"I hate having nobody here, I'd like to know where they all are": Can qualitative research detect differences in Quality of Life among Nursing Home Residents with different levels of Cognitive Impairment?', *Ageing and Mental Health*, 15 (5), 562–572.

Cahill, S., and Shapiro, M. (1993). '"I think he might have hit me once": Aggression towards caregivers in dementia care', *Australian Journal on Ageing*, 12 (4), 10–15.

Cahill, S., and Shapiro, M. (1997). 'At first I thought it was age, family carers' recognition and general practitioners diagnosis of dementia', *New Doctor-Sydney*, 19–23.

Cahill, S., Clark, M., Walsh, C., O'Connell, H., and Lawlor, B. (2006). 'Dementia in primary care: The first survey of Irish general practitioners', *International Journal of Geriatric Psychiatry*, 21 (4), 319–324.

Cahill, S., Diaz-Ponce, A. M., Coen, R. F., and Walsh, C. (2010). 'The under-detection of cognitive impairment in nursing homes in the Dublin area. The need for on-going cognitive assessment', *Age and Ageing*, 39 (1), 128–131.

Cahill, S., O'Shea, E., and Pierce, M. (2012). 'Creating excellence in dementia care: A research review for Ireland's national dementia strategy', *DSIDC's Living with Dementia Research Programme*, School of Social Work and Social Policy, Trinity College, Dublin Irish Centre for Social Gerontology, National University of Ireland, Galway.

Cahill, S., Pierce, M., and Bobersky, A. (2014a). 'An evaluation report on the dementia support worker initiative of the 5 steps to living well with dementia in South Tipperary Project', Genio, Ireland.

Cahill, S., Pierce, M., and Moore, V. (2014b). 'A national survey of memory clinics in the Republic of Ireland', *International Psychogeriatrics*, 26 (4), 605–613.

Cahill, S., O'Nolan, C., O'Caheny, D., and Bobersky, A. (2015a). *An Irish national survey of dementia in long-term residential care*. Dublin: Dementia Services Information and Development Centre, <http://www.dementia.ie/images/uploads/site-images/DSIDCReport_439721.pdf>, accessed 8 April 2020.

Cahill, S., Pierce, M., Werner, P., Darley, A., & Bobersky, A. (2015b). 'A systematic review of the public's knowledge and understanding of Alzheimer's disease and dementia', *Alzheimer Disease & Associated Disorders*, 29(3), 255–275.

Calkins, M. P. (1988). *Design for dementia*. National Health Pub. ISBN: 0932500935.

Caron, C. D., Ducharme, F., and Griffith, J. (2006). 'Deciding on institutionalization for a relative with dementia: The most difficult decision for caregivers', *Canadian Journal on Aging/La Revue canadienne du vieillissement*, 25 (2), 193–205.

Cepoiu-Martin, M., Tam-Tham, H., Patten, S., Maxwell, C. J., and Hogan, D. B. (2016). 'Predictors of long-term care placement in persons with dementia: A systematic review and meta-analysis', *International Journal of Geriatric Psychiatry*, 31 (11), 1151–1171.

Cheng, S. T. (2017). 'Dementia caregiver burden: A research update and critical analysis', *Current Psychiatry Reports*, 19 (9), 64.

Citizens' Assembly. (2017). 'Second report and recommendations of the Citizens' Assembly: How we best respond to the challenges and opportunities of ageing population', <https://www.citizensassembly.ie/en/how-we-best-respond-to-challenges-and-opportunities-of-an-ageing-population/final-report-on-how-we-best-respond-to-the-challenges-and-opportunities-of-an-ageing-population/final-report-on-older-people-incl-appendix-a-d.pdf>, accessed 8 April 2020.

Clare, L. (2002). 'Developing awareness about awareness in early-stage dementia: The role of psychosocial factors', *Dementia*, 1 (3), 295–312.

Clare, L. (2017). 'Rehabilitation for people living with dementia: A practical framework of positive support', *PloS Medicine*, 14 (3).

Clare, L., and Woods, R. T. (2004). 'Cognitive training and cognitive rehabilitation for people with early-stage Alzheimer's disease: A review', *Neuropsychological Rehabilitation*, 14, 385–401.

Clare, L., Bayer, A., Burns, A., Corbett, A., Jones, R., Knapp, M., Kopelman, M., Kudlicka, A., Leroi, I., Oyebode, J., Pool, J., Woods, B., and Whitaker, R. (2013). 'Goal-oriented cognitive rehabilitation in early-stage dementia: Study protocol for a multi-centre single-blind randomised controlled trial (GREAT)', *Trials*, 14 (1), 152.

Clare, L., Kudlicka, A., Oyebode, J. R., Jones, R. W., Bayer, A., Leroi, I., Kopelman, M., James, I. A., Culverwell, A., Pool, J., Brand, A., Henderson, C., Hoare, Z., Knapp, M., Morgan-Trimmer, S., Burns, A., Corbett, A., Whitaker, R., and Woods, B. (2019). 'Goal-oriented cognitive rehabilitation for early-stage Alzheimer's and related dementias: The GREAT RCT', *Health Technology Assessment*, 23 (10).

Clarke, C. L., Keyes, S. E., Wilkinson, H., Alexjuk, J., Wilcockson, J., Robinson, L., Reynolds, J., McClelland, S., Hodgson, Corner, L., and Cattan, M. (2013). 'Healthbridge, The National Evaluation of Peer Support Networks and Dementia Advisers in implementation of the National Dementia Strategy for England [Ref: 025/0058]', Department of Health Policy Research Programme Project.

Code of Practice for Nursing Homes. (1995). *Department of Health and Children*, Dublin, <https://www.lenus.ie/bitstream/handle/10147/46681/1724.pdf?sequence=1&isAllowed=y>

References

Coffey, A., Cornally, N., Hegarty, J., O'Caoimh, R., O'Reilly, P., O'Loughlin, C., Drennan, J., Clarke, C., and Hartigan, I. (2018). 'Evaluation of The Alzheimer Society of Ireland Dementia Adviser Service Report', <https://www.lenus.ie/handle/10147/623818>, accessed 8 April 2020.

Cohen, D., and Eisdorfer, C. (1986). *The loss of self: A family resource for the care of Alzheimer''s disease disorders*. New York and London: W. W. Norton.

Connolly, S., and O'Shea, E. (2015). 'The impact of dementia on length of stay in acute hospitals in Ireland', *Dementia*, 14 (5), 650–658.

Connolly, S., Gillespie, P., O'Shea, E., Cahill, S., and Pierce, M. (2014). 'Estimating the economic and social costs of dementia in Ireland', *Dementia*, 13 (1), 5–22.

Convery, J. (2014). *Here today gone tomorrow: An exploratory study of Housing with Care development for people with dementia in Ireland* (unpublished PhD thesis), Trinity College Dublin, Ireland.

Corrada, M. M., Berlau, D. J., and Kawas, C. H. (2012). 'A population-based clinicopathological study in the oldest-old: The 90+ study', *Current Alzheimer Research*, 9 (6), 709–717.

CRPD. (2006). 'Convention on the Rights of Persons with Disabilities'. Resolution adopted by United Nations, <https://www.un.org/development/desa/disabilities/resources/general-assembly/convention-on-the-rights-of-persons-with-disabilities-ares61106.html>, accessed 8 April 2020.

CSO. (2016). *Census 2016 Reports*. Cork: Central Statistics Office, Ireland.

CSO. (2017). *Population and Labour force Projections 2017–2051*. Cork: Central Statistics Office, Ireland.

Cushman & Wakefield. (2017). *Irish Nursing Home Market 2016/17*. Dublin: Sherry Fitzgerald.

Daatland, S. O., Høyland, K., and Otnes, B. (2015). 'Scandinavian contrasts and Norwegian variations in special housing for older people', *Journal of Housing for the Elderly*, 29 (1–2), 180–196.

DAI. (2016). 'The Human Rights of People Living with Dementia: From Rhetoric to Reality', *Dementia Alliance International*, <http://www.alzheimers.org.nz/getattachment/News-Info/Global-information/Human-Rights-for-People-Living-with-Dementia-Rhetoric-to-Reality.pdf/>, accessed 8 April 2020.

Daly, M. (2018). *ESPN Thematic Report on Challenges in long-term care Ireland*. Brussels: General for Employment, Social Affairs and Inclusion, European Commission.

Davis, B., and Pope, C. (2010). 'Institutionalised ghosting: Policy contexts and language use in erasing the person with Alzheimer's', *Language Policy*, 9 (1), 29–44.

De Lange, J., Willemse, B., Smit, D., and Pot, A. M. (2011). 'Housing with care for people with dementia in the Netherlands' [Powerpoint slides], <http://

www.socialwork-socialpolicy.tcd.ie/livingwithdementia/assets/pdf/JacominedeLange.pdf>, accessed 11 November 2011.

De Lepeleire, J., Wind, A. W., Iliffe, S., Moniz-Cook, E. D., Wilcock, J., González, W. M., Derksen, E., Gianelli, M. V., Vernooij-Dassen, M., and the Interdem Group (2008). 'The primary care diagnosis of dementia in Europe: An analysis using multidisciplinary, multinational expert groups', *Aging and Mental Health*, 12 (5), 568–576.

De Rooij, A. H., Luijkx, K. G., Declercq, A. G., and Schols, J. M. (2011). 'Quality of life of residents with dementia in long-term care settings in the Netherlands and Belgium: Design of a longitudinal comparative study in traditional nursing homes and small-scale living facilities', *BMC Geriatrics*, 11 (1), 20.

De Siún, A. (2013). 'Briefing paper on dementia advisors', *Genio*, <https://www.genio.ie/system/files/publications/GENIO_DEMENTIA_ADVISORS_BP_NO.2.pdf>, accessed 8 April 2020.

De Siún, A., and Guiry, R. (2018). 'Implementing the "Dementia: Understanding Together" National public Awareness campaign in Ireland. Paper presented at Alzheimer Europe Annual Conference in Barcelona, October 29th, <https://www.alzheimer-europe.org/Conferences/Previous-conferences/2018-Barcelona/Detailed-programme-abstracts-and-presentations/(language)/eng-GB>, accessed 8 April 2020.

Degener, T. (2014). *A human rights model of disability*, Routledge Handbook of Disability Law and Human Rights.

Dempsey, C., Normand, C., and Timonen, V. (2016). 'Towards a more person-centred home care service: A study of the preferences of older adults and home care workers', *Administration*, 64 (2), 109–136.

Department of Public Expenditure and Reform. (2018). *Spending Review 2018, Trends in public social care service provision and expenditures for older persons*. Ireland: IGEES, Department of Public Expenditure and Reform, <https://assets.gov.ie/3815/051218171839-b6ba3671cf39468eb4a8b3e3db577a9a.pdf>, accessed 8 April 2020.

Dewing, J. (2008). 'Personhood and dementia: Revisiting Tom Kitwood's ideas', *International Journal of Older People Nursing*, 3 (1), 3–13.

Dhedhi, S. A., Swinglehurst, D., and Russell, J. (2014). "'Timely' diagnosis of dementia: What does it mean? A narrative analysis of GPs' accounts', *BMJ Open*, 4 (3), e004439.

Diaz-Ponce, A. (2014). *Quality of life and anti-dementia medication: An exploration of the experiences of people living with dementia and their care-partners* (unpublished PhD thesis), Trinity College Dublin, Ireland.

DOH. (1995). *Guide to nursing home regulation*. Dublin: Department of Health, Ireland, <https://www.lenus.ie/bitstream/handle/10147/251578/GuideTo

References

TheNursingHomeLegislation.pdf?sequence=1&isAllowed=y>, accessed 8 April 2020.

DOH. (2013). *National positive ageing strategy*. Dublin: Government of Ireland, <https://www.gov.ie/en/publication/737780-national-positive-ageing-strategy/>, accessed 8 April 2020.

DOH. (2014). *The Irish national dementia strategy*. Dublin: Government of Ireland, <https://assets.gov.ie/10870/3276adf5273f4a9aa67e7f3a970d9cb1.pdf>, accessed 8 April 2020.

DOH. (2015). *Review of the nursing homes support scheme: A fair deal*. Dublin: Government of Ireland, <https://assets.gov.ie/14095/f39a443d0a054c78a548d5fad8711df4.pdf>, accessed 8 April 2020.

DOH. (2018). *Health in Ireland: Key trends 2018*. Dublin: Government of Ireland, <https://assets.gov.ie/9441/e5c5417ee4c544b384c262f99da77122.pdf>, accessed 8 April 2020.

DOHC. (1994). *Shaping a healthier future: A strategy for effective health care in the 1990's*. Dublin: Department of Health and Children. Stationary Office.

DOHC. (2001). Quality and fairness. A health system for you. Dublin: Department of Health and Children. Stationary Office.

Donnelly, M. (2019). 'Deciding in dementia: The possibilities and limits of supported decision-making', *International Journal of Law and Psychiatry*, 66, 101466.

Donnelly, S., Cahill, S., and O'Neill, D. (2018). 'Care planning meetings: Issues for policy, multi-disciplinary practice and patient participation', *Practice*, 30 (1), 53–71.

Donnelly, S., O' Brien, M., Begley, E., and Brennan, J. (2016). *I'd prefer to stay at home but I don't have a choice' Meeting Older People's Preference for Care: Policy, but what about practice?* Dublin: University College Dublin.

Dubois, B., Feldman, H. H., Jacova, C., Cummings, J. L., DeKosky, S. T., Barberger-Gateau, P., Delacourte, A., Frisoni, G., Fox, N. C., Galasko, D., Gauthier, S., Hampel H., Jicha, G. A., Meguro, K., O'Brien, J., Pasquier, F., Robert, P., Rossor, M., Salloway, S. Sarazin, M., de Souza, L. C., Stern, Y., Visser, P. J., and Scheltens, P. (2010). 'Revising the definition of Alzheimer's disease: A new lexicon', *The Lancet Neurology*, 9 (11), 1118–1127.

Eastwood, M. (1994). 'Abnormal behaviour associated with dementia', *International Psychiatry Today*, 4, 8–10.

EDJN. (2019). 'The EU might well achieve its employment rate target for 2020', *European Data Journalism Network*, <https://www.europeandatajournalism.eu/eng/News/Data-news/The-EU-might-well-achieve-its-employment-rate-target-for-2020>, accessed 8 April 2020.

Eisdorfer, C. E., and Lawton, M. (1973). *The psychology of adult development and aging*. American Psychological Association.

Etters, L., Goodall, D., and Harrison, B. E. (2008). 'Caregiver burden among dementia patient caregivers: A review of the literature', *Journal of the American Academy of Nurse Practitioners*, 20 (8), 423–428.

Eurobarometer, S. (2007). 'Health and long-term care in the European Union', *Special Eurobarometer*, 283.

Eurostat. (2018). 'Population structure and aging', <https://ec.europa.eu/eurostat/statistics-explained/index.php/Population_structure_and_ageing>, accessed 8 April 2020.

Family Carers Ireland. (2017). 'Carers and Employment: Socioeconomic data from the 2011 and 2016, Irish Censuses', *Family Carers Ireland*, <https://familycarers.ie/wp-content/uploads/2017/11/Carers-and-Employment-Data-from-the-2011-and-2016-Irish-Censuses.pdf>, accessed 8 April 2020.

Family Carers Ireland. (2019). 'Paying the price', *Family Carers Ireland*, College of Psychiatrists of Ireland, UCD School of Nursing, Midwifery & Health Systems, <https://familycarers.ie/wp-content/uploads/2019/05/Paying-the-Price-The-Physical-Mental-and-Psychological-Impact-of-Caring.pdf>, accessed 8 April 2020.

Fang, R., Ye, S., Huangfu, J., and Calimag, D. P. (2017). 'Music therapy is a potential intervention for cognition of Alzheimer's disease: A mini-review', *Translational Neurodegeneration*, 6 (1), 2.

Flynn, E. (2018). 'Legal capacity for people with dementia: A human rights approach'. In S. Cahill (ed.), *Dementia and Human Rights*, 157–174. Bristol: Policy Press.

Flynn, E., and Arstein-Kerslake, A. (2014). 'Legislating personhood: Realising the right to support in exercising legal capacity', *International Journal of Law in Context*, 10 (1), 81–104.

Foley, T. (2017). *The design, development and evaluation of dementia training for General Practitioners*, Thesis submitted to the College of Medicine and Health, National University of Ireland, Cork.

Foley, T., Jennings, A., and Swanwick, G. (2019). 'Dementia: Diagnosis & management in general practice – Quick reference guide. Quality and safety in practice committee', *ICGP*, <http://dementiapathways.ie/_filecache/e74/e54/839-dementia_qrg_15th_april_2019-1.pdf>, accessed 8 April 2020.

Fortinsky, R. H., Tennen, H., and Steffens, D. C. (2013). 'Resilience in the face of chronic illness and family caregiving in middle and later life', *Psychiatric Annals*, 43 (12), 549–554.

Fossey, J. (2010). 'Care homes'. In M. Downs and B. Bowers (eds), *Excellence in dementia care: Research into practice*, 336–358. McGraw-Hill Education (UK).

References

Fox, S., Cahill, S., McGown, R and Kilty, C. (2020). *A review of diagnostic and post-diagnostic processes and pathways for people living with young-onset dementia*. HSE.

Fratiglioni, L., and Wang, H. X. (2007). 'Brain reserve hypothesis in dementia', *Journal of Alzheimer's Disease*, 12 (1), 11–22.

Gaugler, J. E., Davey, A., Pearlin, L. I., and Zarit, S. H. (2000). 'Modeling caregiver adaptation over time: The longitudinal impact of behavior problems', *Psychology and Aging*, 15 (3), 437.

Gaugler, J. E., Duval, S., Anderson, K. A., and Kane, R. L. (2007). 'Predicting nursing home admission in the US: A meta-analysis', *BMC Geriatrics*, 7 (1), 13.

Genet, N., Boerma, W., Kroneman, M., Hutchinson, A., and Saltman, R. B. (2012). *Home care across Europe, The European observatory on health systems and policies*, Observatory Studies Series, 27. Brussels: WHO European Centre for Health Policy, 2–5.

George, D. R. (2010). 'Overcoming the social death of dementia through language', *The Lancet*, 76 (9741), 586–587.

George, L., and Gwyther, L. (1986). 'Caregiver well-being: A multidimensional examination of family caregivers of demented adults', *The Gerontologist*, 26, 253–259.

Giaccone, G., Arzberger, T., Alafuzoff, I., Al-Sarraj, S., Budka, H., Duyckaerts, C., Falkai, P., Ironside, J. W., Kovács, G. G., Meyronet, D., Parchi, P., Patsouris, E., Revesz, T., Riederer, P., Rozemuller, A, Schmitt, A., Winblad, B., Kretzschmar, H. (2011). 'New lexicon and criteria for the diagnosis of Alzheimer's disease', *The Lancet Neurology*, 10(4), 298–299.

Gillespie, P., O'Shea, E., Cullinan, J., Lacey, L., Gallagher, D., Ni Mhaolain, A., and Lawlor, B for the Enhancing Care in Alzheimer's Disease (ECAD) Study Team. (2013). 'The effects of dependence and function on costs of care for Alzheimer's disease and mild cognitive impairment in Ireland', *International Journal of Geriatric Psychiatry*, 28 (3), 256–264.

Gilliard, J., and Marshall, M. (2012). *Transforming the quality of life for people with dementia through contact with the natural world: Fresh air on my face*. London and Philadelphia: Jessica Kingsley Publishers.

Gilliard, J., Means, R., Beattie, A., and Daker-White, G. (2005). 'Dementia care in England and the social model for disability-lessons and issues', *Dementia, the International Journal of Social Research and Practice*, 4 (4), 571–586.

Gilmour, J. A., and Brannelly, T. (2010). 'Representations of people with dementia-subaltern, person, citizen', *Nursing Inquiry*, 17 (3), 240–247.

Gilsenan, A. (2010). *The Irish Times*, September 28th.

Glendinning, C. (2018). 'Peer Review on improving reconciliation of work and long-term care: Combining paid work and family care; the impacts of care leave and other measures to improve work-life balance'. *DG Employment, Social Affairs and Inclusion*, European Commission.

Glynn, R. W., Shelley, E., and Lawlor, B. A. (2017). 'Public knowledge and understanding of dementia – evidence from a national survey in Ireland', *Age and Ageing*, 46 (5), 865–869.

Górska, S., Forsyth, K., and Maciver, D. (2018). 'Living with dementia: A meta-synthesis of qualitative research on the lived experience', *The Gerontologist*, 58 (3), e180-e196.

Gove, D., Downs, M., Vernooij-Dassen, M., and Small, N. (2015). 'Stigma and GPs' perceptions of dementia', *Aging and Mental Health*, 20 (4), 1–10.

Hayo, H., Ward, A., and Parkes, J. (2018). *Young-onset dementia: A guide to recognition, diagnosis, and supporting individuals with dementia and their families.* Jessica Kingsley Publishers.

Hanly, P., and Sheerin, C. (2017). 'Valuing informal care in Ireland: Beyond the traditional production boundary', *The Economic and Social Review*, 48 (3, Autumn), 337–364.

Health (Nursing Home) Act. (1990). *Office of Attorney General*, Dublin, <http://www.irishstatutebook.ie/eli/1990/act/23/enacted/en/html>

Health Act. (2007). *Office of Attorney General*, Dublin, <http://www.irishstatutebook.ie/eli/2007/act/23/enacted/en/print>

Heggestad, A. K. T., Nortvedt, P., and Slettebø, Å. (2015). 'Dignity and care for people with dementia living in nursing homes', *Dementia*, 14 (6), 825–841.

Heintz, H., Monette, P., Epstein-Lubow, G., Smith, L., Rowlett, S., and Forester, B. P. (2020). 'Emerging collaborative care models for dementia care in the primary care setting: A narrative review', *The American Journal of Geriatric Psychiatry*, 28 (3), 320–330.

Hennelly, N., Cooney, A., Houghton, C., and O'Shea, E. (2018). 'The experiences and perceptions of personhood for people living with dementia: A qualitative evidence synthesis protocol', *HRB Open Research*, 1 (18), 18.

Hennelly, N., Cooney, A., Houghton, C., and O'Shea, E. (2019). 'Personhood and dementia care: A qualitative evidence synthesis of the perspectives of people with dementia', *The Gerontologist*.

Higgs, P., and Gilleard, C. (2016). 'Interrogating personhood and dementia', *Aging & Mental Health*, 20 (8), 773–780.

HIQA. (2009). *National quality standards for residential care settings for older people in Ireland.* Ireland: Health Information Quality Authority, <https://www.lenus.ie/bitstream/handle/10147/76688/Natqualitystandresidcare.pdf?sequence=1&isAllowed=y>, accessed 8 April 2020.

HIQA. (2016). *Overview report of disability inspections.* Ireland: Health Information Quality Authority, <https://www.hiqa.ie/hiqa-news-updates/hiqa-publishes-overview-report-disability-inspections>, accessed 8 April 2020.

Hoff, A., Reichert, M., Hamblin, K. A., Perek-Bialas, J., and Principi, A. (2014). 'Informal and formal reconciliation strategies of older peoples' working carers: The European carers@ work project', *Vulnerable Groups & Inclusion*, 5 (1), 24264.

Horttana, B. M., Ahlström, G., and Fahlström, G. (2007). 'Patterns of and reasons for relocation in dementia care', *Geriatric Nursing*, 28 (3), 193–200.

Hourihan, A. (2018). Anne Marie Hourihan, *Times Ireland*, 14 July.

HSE (2018). *Mid-term review of the implementation of the national dementia strategy*. Government of Ireland.

Hughes, J. (2011). *Thinking through dementia: International perspectives in philosophy and psychiatry*. Oxford: Oxford University Press.

Hughes, J. (2014). *How we think about dementia: Personhood, rights ethics, the arts and what they mean for care*. London: Jessica Kingsley Publishers.

Hung, L., and Chaudhury, H. (2011). 'Exploring personhood in dining experiences of residents with dementia in long-term care facilities', *Journal of Aging Studies*, 25 (1), 1 12.

Hutchinson, K., Roberts, C., Daly, M., Bulsara, C., and Kurrle, S. (2016). 'E'mpowerment of young people who have a parent living with dementia: A social model perspective', *International Psychogeriatrics*, 28 (4), 657–668.

Iliffe, S., Robinson, L., Brayne, C., Goodman, C., Rait, G., Manthorpe, J., and Ashley, P. (2009). 'Primary care and dementia: 1. Diagnosis, screening and disclosure', *International Journal of Geriatric Psychiatry*, 24 (9), 895–901.

Innes, A. (2009). *Dementia studies*. London: Sage.

Ireland Nursing Home. (2014). 'Health's Ageing Crisis: Time for Action', *BDO*, <https://www.bdo.ie/en-gb/insights/advisory/consulting/health-s-ageing-crisis-time-for-action>, accessed 8 April 2020.

Jack Jr, C. R., Albert, M. S., Knopman, D. S., McKhann, G. M., Sperling, R. A., Carrillo, M. C., Thies, B., and Phelps, C. H. (2011). 'Introduction to the recommendations from the National Institute on Aging-Alzheimer's Association workgroups on diagnostic guidelines for Alzheimer's disease', *Alzheimer's & Dementia*, 7 (3), 257–262.

Jack Jr, C. R., Wiste, H. J., Schwarz, C. G., Lowe, V. J., Senjem, M. L., Vemuri, P., Weigand, S. D., Therneau, T. M., Knopman, D. S. Gunter, J. L., Jones, D. T., Graff-Radford, J., Kantarci, K., Roberts, R. O., Mielke, M. M., Machulda, M. M., and Petersen, R. C. (2018). 'Longitudinal tau PET in ageing and Alzheimer's disease', *Brain*, 141 (5), 1517–1528.

Jefferies, K., and Agrawal, N. (2009). 'Early-onset dementia', *Advances in Psychiatric Treatment*, 15 (5), 380–388.

Kahn, R. L. (1975). 'The mental health system and the future aged', *The Gerontologist*, 15 (1_Part_2), 24–31.

Kane, R. A. (2001). 'Long-term care and a good quality of life: Bringing them closer together', *The Gerontologist*, 41 (3), 293–304.

Keady, J., Ashcroft-Simpson, S., Halligan, K., and Williams, S. (2007). 'Admiral nursing and the family care of a parent with dementia: Using autobiographical narrative as grounding for negotiated clinical practice and decision-making', *Scandinavian Journal of Caring Sciences*, 21 (3), 345–353.

Kelley, B. J., Boeve, B. F., and Josephs, K. A. (2008). 'Young-onset dementia: Demographic and etiologic characteristics of 235 patients', *Archives of Neurology*, 65 (11), 1502–1508.

Kelly, M. E., and O'Sullivan, M. (2015). 'Strategies and techniques for cognitive rehabilitation; manual for healthcare professionals working with people with cognitive impairment', *Trinity College Dublin, NEIL & The Alzheimer Society of Ireland*, <https://www.researchgate.net/profile/Michelle_Kelly8/publication/282910314_Strategies_and_Techniques_for_Cognitive_Rehabilitation_Manual_for_Healthcare_Professionals_Working_with_Individuals_with_Cognitive_Impairment/links/562240b308ae93a5c927e752.pdf>, accessed 8 April 2020.

Kelly, M. E., Finan, S., Lawless, M., Scully, N., Fitzpatrick, J., Quigley, M., Tyrrell, F., O'Regan, A., and Devane, A. (2017). 'An evaluation of community-based cognitive stimulation therapy: A pilot study with an Irish population of people with dementia', *Irish Journal of Psychological Medicine*, 34 (3), 157–167.

Keogh, F., Pierce, M., and O'Shea, E. (2019). *Ageing, social care & social justice: Policy Symposium proceedings*. Centre for Economic and Social Research on Dementia. NUI Galway.

Keogh, F., Pierce, M., Neylon, K., and Fleming, P. (2018a). 'Intensive home care packages for people with dementia: A realist evaluation protocol', *BMC Health Services Research*, 18 (1), 829.

Keogh, F., Pierce, M., Neylon, K., Fleming, P., O'Neill, S., Carter, L., & O'Shea, E. (2018b). *Supporting older people with complex needs at home: What works for people with dementia*. Dublin: Genio.

Kim S. (2015). 'Cognitive rehabilitation for elderly people with early-stage Alzheimer's disease', *Journal of Physical Therapy Science*, 27, 543–546.

Kittay, E. F. (2007). 'Beyond autonomy and paternalism: The caring transparent self. Autonomy and paternalism', *Reflections on the Theory and Practice of Health Care*, 23–70.

Kitwood, T. (1990). 'The dialectics of dementia: With particular reference to Alzheimer's disease', *Ageing and Society*, 10 (2), 177–196.

Kitwood, T. (1993a). 'Person and process in dementia', *International Journal of Geriatric Psychiatry*, 8, 541–555.

Kitwood, T. (1993b). 'Towards a theory of dementia care: The interpersonal process', *Ageing and Society*, 13 (1), 51–67.

Kitwood, T. (1995). 'Positive long-term changes in dementia: Some preliminary observations', *Journal of Mental Health*, 4 (2), 133–144.

Kitwood, T. (1997a). *Dementia reconsidered: The person comes first.* Buckingham: Open University Press.

Kitwood, T. (1997b). 'The experience of dementia', *Aging & Mental Health*, 1 (1), 13–22.

Kitwood, T., and Bredin, K. (1992). 'Towards a theory of dementia care: Personhood and well-being', *Ageing & Society*, 12 (3), 269–287.

Knapp, M., Comas-Herrera, A., Somani, A., and Banerjee, S. (2007). 'Dementia: International comparisons'. *LSE/PSSRU, Institute of Psychiatry at the Maudsley*, London School of Economics and Political Science.

Knapp, M., Thorgrimsen, L., Patel, A., Spector, A., Hallam, A., Woods, B., and Orrell, M. (2006). 'Cognitive stimulation therapy for people with dementia: Cost-effectiveness analysis', *The British Journal of Psychiatry*, 188 (6), 574–580.

Koopmans, R., and Rosness, T. (2014). 'Young-onset dementia – what does the name imply?', *International Psychogeriatrics*, 26 (12), 1931–1933.

Krishnamoorthy, A., and Anderson, D. (2011). 'Managing challenging behaviour in older adults with dementia', *Progress in Neurology and Psychiatry*, 15 (3), 20–26.

Lafferty, A., Fealy, G., Downes, C., and Drennan, J. (2014). 'Family carers of older people: Results of a National Survey of Stress'. *Conflict and Coping* [Internet]. Belfield: University College Dublin.

Lafferty, A., Fealy, G., Teahan, A., McAuliffe, E., Phelan, A., O'Sullivan, L., and O'Shea, D. (2016). 'Profiling family carers of people with dementia: Results from a national survey'. *Poster presentation at the Irish Gerontological Society annual conference*, Killarney, September 2016.

Larkin, M., and Milne, A. (2017). 'What do we know about older former carers? Key issues and themes', *Health & Social Care in the Community*, 25 (4), 1396–1403.

Lawlor, B., and Brennan, S. (2016). *A pocket positive guide to dementia.* Dublin: Trinity Brain Health.

Lawton, M. P. (2001). 'The physical environment of the person with Alzheimer's disease', *Aging & Mental Health*, 5 (sup1), 56–64.

Lawton, M. P., Van Haitsma, K., and Klapper, J. (1996). 'Observed affect in nursing home residents with Alzheimer's disease', *The Journals of Gerontology Series B: Psychological Sciences and Social Sciences*, 51 (1), P3–P14.

Lawton, M. P., Van Haitsma, K., Perkinson, M., and Ruckdeschel, K. (1999). 'Observed affect and quality of life in dementia: Further affirmations and problems', *Journal of Mental Health and Aging*, 5 (1), 69–81.

Lawton, M. P., Weisman, G. D., Sloane, P., and Calkins, M. (1997). 'Assessing environments for older people with chronic illness', *Journal of Mental Health and Ageing*, 3, 83–100.

Lazarus, R. S., and Folkman, S. (1984). *Stress, appraisal, and coping.* Springer.

Lindemann, H. (2014). 'Second nature and tragedy of Alzheimer's'. In L.-C. Hydén, H. Lindemann and J. Brookmeier (eds), *Beyond loss: Dementia, identity, personhood*, 11–23. Oxford Scholarship Online, Oxford University Press.

Livingston, G., Sommerlad, A., Orgeta, V., Costafreda, S. G., Huntley, J., Ames, D., Clive Ballard, C., Banerjee, S., Burns, A., Cohen-Mansfield, J., Cooper, C., Fox, N., Gitlin, L. N., Howard, R., Kales, H. C., Larson, E. B., Ritchie, K., Rockwood, K., Sampson, E. L., Samus, Q., Schneider, L. S., Selbæk, G., Linda Teri, L., and Mukadam, N. (2017). 'Dementia prevention, intervention, and care', *The Lancet*, 390 (10113), 2673–2734.

Livingston, G., Huntley, J., Sommerlad, A., Ames, D., Ballard, C., Banerjee, S., Brayne, C., Burns, A., Cohen-Mansfield, J., Cooper, C., and Costafreda, S. G. (2020). Dementia prevention, intervention, and care: 2020 report of the Lancet Commission. *The Lancet*, *396*(10248), 413–446.

Luengo-Fernandez, R., Leal, J., and Gray, A. (2010). 'Dementia 2010: The economic burden of dementia and associated research funding in the United Kingdom', *Alzheimer's Research Trust*, Health Economics Research Centre, University of Oxford, <https://www.alzheimersresearchuk.org/wp-content/uploads/2015/01/Dementia2010Full.pdf>, accessed 8 April 2020.

Luppa, M., Luck, T., Weyerer, S., König, H. H., Brähler, E., and Riedel-Heller, S. G. (2010). 'Prediction of institutionalization in the elderly, A systematic review', *Age and Ageing*, 39 (1), 31–38.

Malmberg, B., and Zarit, S. H. (1993). 'Group homes for people with dementia: A Swedish example', *The Gerontologist*, 33 (5), 682–686.

Matsuda, O. (1999). 'Reliability and validity of the subjective burden scale in family caregivers of elderly relatives with dementia', *International Psychogeriatrics*, 11 (2), 159–170.

Matthews, F. E., Stephan, B. C., Robinson, L., Jagger, C., Barnes, L. E., Arthur, A., and Brayne, C. (2016). 'A two decade dementia incidence comparison from the Cognitive Function and Ageing Studies I and II', *Nature Communications*, 7 (1), 1–8.

Mayrhofer, A., Mathie, E., McKeown, J., Bunn, F. and Goodman, C. (2018) 'Age-appropriate services for people diagnosed with young-onset dementia (YOD): A systematic review', *Aging & Mental Health*, 22 (8), 933–941.

McCormack, B. (2001). 'Autonomy and the relationship between nurses and older people', *Ageing & Society*, 21 (4), 417–446.

McCormack, B. (2004). 'Person-centredness in gerontological nursing: An overview of the literature', *Journal of Clinical Nursing*, 13, 31–38.

McCormack, B., Roberts, T., Meyer, J., Morgan, D., and Boscart, V. (2012). 'Appreciating the 'person' in long-term care', *International Journal of Older People Nursing*, 7 (4), 284–294.

McKhann, G. M., Knopman, D. S., Chertkow, H., Hyman, B. T., Jack Jr, C. R., Kawas, C. H., Klunk, W. E., Koroshetz, W. J., Manly, J. J., Mayeux, R., Mohs, R. C., Morris, J. C., Rossor, M. N., Scheltens, P., Carrillo, M. C., Thies, B., Weintraub, S., and Phelps, C. H. (2011). 'The diagnosis of dementia due to Alzheimer's disease: Recommendations from the National Institute on Aging-Alzheimer's Association workgroups on diagnostic guidelines for Alzheimer's disease', *Alzheimer's & Dementia*, 7 (3), 263–269.

McLean, A. (2010). 'New approaches to nursing home/dementia care in the US: A contextual review', *Paper presented at Living with Dementia Seminar*, Long Room Hub, Trinity College Dublin, Sept 29th.

Mental Health Foundation. (2015). *Dementia rights and the social model of disability: A new direction for policy and practice*. London: Mental Health Foundation.

Milne, A. (2010). 'The 'D'word: Reflections on the relationship between stigma, discrimination and dementia', *Journal of Mental Health*, 19 (3), 227–233.

Milne, A., Guss, R., and Russ, A. (2014). 'Psycho-educational support for relatives of people with a recent diagnosis of mild to moderate dementia: An evaluation of a "Course for Carers"', *Dementia*, 13 (6), 768–787.

Mishra, V., and Barrett, J. (2016). *Reablement and older people*. IFA Copenhagen Summit.

Mormont, E., Jamart, J., and Jacques, D. (2014). 'Symptoms of depression and anxiety after the disclosure of the diagnosis of Alzheimer disease', *Journal of Geriatric Psychiatry and Neurology*, 27 (4), 231–236.

Murphy, K., and Welford, C. (2012). 'Agenda for the future: Enhancing autonomy for older people in residential care', *International Journal of Older People Nursing*, 7 (1), 75–80.

Murray, L. M., and Boyd, S. (2009). 'Protecting personhood and achieving quality of life for older adults with dementia in the US health care system', *Journal of Aging and Health*, 21 (2), 350–373.

National Institute on Ageing. 'Brain health'. *US Department of Health & Human Services*, <https://www.nia.nih.gov/health/topics/brain-health>

Nedlund, A. C., Bartlett, R., and Clarke, C. L. (2019). *Everyday citizenship and people with dementia*. Dunedin Academic Press.

Newhouse, P., and Lasek, J. (2006). 'Assessment and diagnosis of severe dementia', *Severe Dementia*, NJ: John Wiley and Sons, 3–20.

NHSS. (2009). *Nursing Home Support Scheme Act, 15*. Dublin: Office of the Attorney General, Government of Ireland, <http://www.irishstatutebook.ie/eli/2009/act/15/enacted/en/html>, accessed 8 April 2020.

NICE. (2018). 'Dementia Assessment Management and Support for People living with Dementia and their Carers, NG 97'. *National Institute for Health and*

Care Excellence (NICE), <www.nice.org.uk/guidance/ng97>, accessed 8 April 2020.

NICE/SCIE. (2006). *Dementia: A NICE-SCIE guideline on supporting people with dementia and their carers in health and social care*. National Clinical Practice Guideline No. 42. National Institute for Health and Clinical Excellence/Social Care Institute for Excellence, London: NICE/SCIE.

Nolan, L., McCarron, M., McCallion, P., and Murphy-Lawless, J. (2006). 'Perceptions of stigma in dementia: An exploratory study', *Alzheimer Society of Ireland*, <https://www.lenus.ie/bitstream/handle/10147/299918/StigmainDementiaReport.pdf?sequence=1&isAllowed=y>, accessed 8 April 2020.

Nordenfelt, L. (2004). 'The varieties of dignity', *Health Care Analysis*, 12 (2), 69–81; discussion 83–89.

Nuffield Council on Bioethics. (2009). *Dementia: Ethical issues*. London: Nuffield Council on Bioethics.

Nursing Home Act. (1990). *Health Nursing Home Act*. Dublin: Office of the Attorney General, Government of Ireland, <http://www.irishstatutebook.ie/eli/1990/act/23/enacted/en/html>, accessed 8 April 2020.

O'Connor, D., and Purves, B. (2009). *Decision-Making, Personhood and Dementia: Exploring the Interface*. London: Jessica Kingsley Publishers.

OECD. (2015). *Addressing dementia: The OECD response*. OECD Health Policy Studies. Paris: OECD Publishing. <http://dx.doi.org/10.1787/9789264231726-en>, accessed 8 April 2020.

O'Neill, D. (2006). *A review of the deaths at Leas-Cross Nursing Home 2002–2005*. Ireland: Health Service Executive Publications, <https://www.hse.ie/eng/services/publications/olderpeople/leas-cross-report-.pdf>, accessed 8 April 2020.

O'Shea, E. (2003). 'Costs and consequences for the carers of people with dementia in Ireland', *Dementia*, 2 (2), 201–219.

O'Shea, E., and Carney, P. (2017). 'Dementia: Paying dividends. A report on the Atlantic Philanthropies Investment in Dementia in Ireland'. *NUI Galway and Centre for Economic and Social Research on Dementia*, National University of Ireland, Galway.

O'Shea, E., and O'Reilly, S. (1999). *An action plan for dementia*. Dublin: National Council on Ageing and Older People, Ireland.

O'Shea, E., Devane, D., Cooney, A., Casey, D., Jordan, F., Hunter, A., Murphy, E., Newell, J., Connolly, S., and Murphy, K. (2014). 'The impact of reminiscence on the quality of life of residents with dementia in long-stay care', *International Journal of Geriatric Psychiatry*, 29 (10), 1062–1070.

O'Shea, E., Keogh, F., and Heneghan, C. (2018). *Post-diagnostic support for people with dementia and their carers*. Centre for Economic and Social Research on Dementia, NUI Galway.

O'Shea, E., Keogh, F., and Cooney, A. (2019). 'The continuum of care for people living with dementia in Ireland'. *Centre for Economic and Social Research on Dementia*, NUI Galway and National Dementia Office, HSE, Ireland.

Oireachtas Committee on the Future of Health (2017). *Committee on the Future of Health, Sláintecare report*. Dublin: Houses of the Oireachtas, Ireland, <https://www.gov.ie/pdf/?file=https://assets.gov.ie/165/270718095030-1134389-Slaintecare-Report-May-2017.pdf#page=1>, accessed 8 April 2020.

Oliver, M. (1983). *Social work with disabled people*. Basingstoke: Macmillan.

PA Consulting. (2018). *Health Service Capacity Review 2018. Review of Health Demand and Capacity Requirements in Ireland to 2031*. Dublin: Department of Health, Ireland.

Park, M., Butcher, H. K., and Maas, M. L. (2004). 'A thematic analysis of Korean family caregivers' experiences in making the decision to place a family member with dementia in a long-term care facility', *Research in Nursing & Health*, 27 (5), 345–356.

Parsons, T. (2015). *Reminiscence work in four dementia care settings in Ireland: The experience of the person with dementia and the facilitator* (unpublished PhD thesis), Trinity College Dublin, Ireland.

Pearlin, L. I., Mullan, J. T., Semple, S. J., and Skaff, M. M. (1990). 'Caregiving and the stress process: An overview of concepts and their measures', *The Gerontologist*, 30 (5), 583–594.

Pertl, M. M., Hannigan, C., Brennan, S., Robertson, I. H., and Lawlor, B. A. (2017). 'Cognitive reserve and self-efficacy as moderators of the relationship between stress exposure and executive functioning among spousal dementia caregivers', *International Psychogeriatrics*, 29 (4), 615–625.

Pertl, M. M., Sooknarine-Rajpatty, A., Brennan, S., Robertson, I. H., and Lawlor, B. A. (2019). 'Caregiver choice and caregiver outcomes: A longitudinal study of Irish spousal dementia caregivers', *Frontiers in Psychology*, 10.

Pierce, M. (2019). The PREPARED (Primary, Care, Education, Pathways and Research of Dementia) Project. A Synthesis Report.

Pierce, M., and Pierse, T. (eds) (2017). 'Informal caregiving to people with dementia'. In O'Shea, E., Cahill, S., and Pierce, M. (eds), *Developing and implementing policy on dementia in Ireland*, 41–47. Galway: Centre for Economic and Social Research on Dementia in Ireland, National University of Ireland.

Pierce, M., Cahill, S., and O'Shea, E. (2014). 'Prevalence and projections of dementia in Ireland', 2011 report prepared for Genio, Ltd.

Pierse, T., O'Shea, E., and Carney, P. (2019). 'Estimates of the prevalence, incidence and severity of dementia in Ireland', *Irish Journal of Psychological Medicine*, 36 (2), 129–137.

Pierce, M., Keogh, F., Teahan, A., and O'Shea, E. (2019). *Report of an evaluation of the HSE's National Dementia Post-Diagnostic Support Grant Scheme*. Tullamore: National Dementia Office.

Pinquart, M., and Sörensen, S. (2003). 'Differences between caregivers and non-caregivers in psychological health and physical health: A meta-analysis', *Psychology and Aging*, 18 (2), 250.
Post, S. (2000). *The moral challenge of Alzheimer's disease: Ethical issues from diagnosis to dying*. Baltimore, MD: John Hopkins University.
Pot, A. M. (2013). 'Improving nursing home care for dementia: Is the environment the answer?', *Aging & Mental Health*, 17 (7), 785–787.
Pot, A. M., and Petrea, I. (2013). 'Improving dementia care worldwide: Ideas and advice on developing and implementing a National Dementia Plan', *Bupa/ADI*, London. <https://www.alz.co.uk/sites/default/files/pdfs/global-dementia-plan-report-ENGLISH.pdf>, accessed 8 April 2020.
Pot, A. M., and de Lange, J. (2010). *Monitor woonvormen dementie. Een studie naar verpleeghuiszorg voor mensen met dementie*. Trimbos Instituut.
Poulshock, S. W., and Deimling, G. T. (1984). 'Families caring for elders in residence: Issues in the measurement of burden', *Journal of Gerontology*, 39 (2), 230–239.
Prime Time. (2005). *Leas Cross nursing home*. Prime Time Investigates, RTE (Ireland), May 30th.
Prince, M. (2015). 'Paper presented at the inaugural Global Brain Health Institute Conference', December 8–11, 2015. Institute meeting, Havana, Cuba.
Prince, M., Knapp, M., Guerchet, M., McCrone, P., Prina, M., Comas-Herrera, A., Wittenberg, R., Adelaja, B., Hu, B., King, D., Rehill, A., and Salimkumar, D. (2014). *Dementia UK update, second edition*. Alzheimer Society.
Pullman, D. (1999). 'The ethics of autonomy and dignity in long-term care', *Canadian Journal on Aging/La Revue canadienne du vieillissement*, 18 (1), 26–46.
Quinn, G. (2010). 'Personhood & legal capacity: Perspectives on the paradigm shift of Article 12 CRPD', In Conference on Disability and Legal Capacity under the CRPD, Harvard Law School, Boston (20), 3–5.
Qureshi, H., and Walker, A. (1989). *Caring relationship: Family care of elderly people*. Macmillan Education.
Regulation Lunacy Act. (1871). *Regulation Lunacy Act*. Dublin: Stationery Office, Ireland.
Reves, A., Timmons, S., Fox, S., Murphy, A., and O'Shea, E. (2018). *Dementia Diagnostic Services for Ireland: A literature review*. Tullamore: National Dementia Office.
Revolta, C., Orrell, M., and Spector, A. (2016). 'The biopsychosocial (BPS) model of dementia as a tool for clinical practice. A pilot study', *International Psychogeriatrics*, 28 (7), 1079–1089.
Robins, J. (1988). *The years ahead: A policy for the elderly: Report of the Working Party on Services for the Elderly*. Dublin: Stationary Office.

Robinson, A., Eccleston, C., Annear, M., Elliott, K. E., Andrews, S., Stirling, C., Ashby, M., Donohue, C., Banks, S., Toye, C., and McInerney, F. (2014). 'Who knows, who cares? Dementia knowledge among nurses, care workers, and family members of people living with dementia', *Journal of Palliative Care*, 30 (3), 158–165.

Robinson, L., Hutchings, D., Corner, L., Finch, T., Hughes, J., Brittain, K., and Bond, J. (2007). 'Balancing rights and risks: Conflicting perspectives in the management of wandering in dementia', *Health, Risk & Society*, 9 (4), 389–406.

Rochford-Brennan, H. (2019). 'Dementia as a Human Rights Concern'. *A symposium on Dementia and Human Rights organized by the Trinity Medical and Health Humanities Initiative*, Trinity Collage Dublin, November 8th.

Rogers, K., Coleman, H., Brodtmann, A., Darby, D., and Anderson, V. (2017). 'Family members' experience of the pre-diagnostic phase of dementia: A synthesis of qualitative evidence', *International Psychogeriatrics*, 29 (9), 1425–1437.

Rossor, M. N., Fox, N. C., Mummery, C. J., Schott, J. M., and Warren, J. D. (2010). 'The diagnosis of young-onset dementia', *The Lancet Neurology*, 9 (8), 793–806.

Sabat, S. (1994). 'Excess disability and malignant social psychology: A case study of Alzheimer's disease', *Journal of Community & Applied Social Psychology*, 4 (3), 157–166.

Sabat, S. (2005). 'Capacity for decision-making in Alzheimer's disease: Selfhood, positioning and semiotic persons', *Australian and New Zealand Journal of Psychiatry*, 39, 1030–1035.

Sabat, S. (2014). 'Understanding people with Alzheimer's disease: A biopsychosocial approach', *Paper presented at the Genio Conference*, Davenport Hotel, Dublin, December 2014.

Sabat, S. R. (2001). *The experience of Alzheimer's disease: Life through a tangled veil*. Oxford/Malden, MA: Blackwell

Sabat, S. R. (2010). 'Prepositioning, malignant positioning and the disempowering loss of privileges endured by people with Alzheimer's disease'. In D. M. Moghaddam and R. Harré, R. (eds), *Words of conflict, words of war: How the language we use in political processes sparks fighting*, 89–104. USA: ABC-CLIO.

Sabat, S. R. (2018). *Alzheimer's disease and dementia: What everyone needs to know*. Oxford University Press.

Sabat, S. R. (2019). 'Looking beyond pathology: People with dementia can teach us about our shared humanity'. *A symposium on Dementia and Human Rights*. Trinity College Dublin, November 8th.

Sabat, S. R., Johnson, A., Swarbrick, C., and Keady, J. (2011). 'The 'demented other' or simply 'a person'? Extending the philosophical discourse of Naue and Kroll through the situated self', *Nursing Philosophy*, 12 (4), 282–292.

Sage (2018). *Financing Long-term care in Ireland. The need for a transformative policy agenda: A discussion document*. Dublin: Sage Advocacy.

Schulz, R., Belle, S. H., Czaja, S. J., McGinnis, K. A., Stevens, A., and Zhang, S. (2004). 'Long-term care placement of dementia patients and caregiver health and well-being', *Jama*, 292 (8), 961–967.

SCIE. (2014). 'Useful links for Dementia'. Social Care Institute for Excellence, <https://www.scie.org.uk/dementia/resources/dementia-links.asp>, accessed 8 April 2020.

Seetharaman, K., and Chaudhury, H. (2020). 'I am making a difference': Understanding advocacy as a citizenship practice among persons living with dementia', *Journal of Aging Studies*, 52, 100831.

Shanahan, C. (2019). 'Pricing review of the nursing home fee structure to be published', *Irish Examiner*, 14 November, <https://www.irishexaminer.com/breakingnews/ireland/pricing-review-of-the-nursing-home-fee-structure-to-be-published-964247.html>, accessed 8April 2020.

Sharma, N., Chakrabarti, S., and Grover, S. (2016). 'Gender differences in caregiving among family-caregivers of people with mental illnesses', *World Journal of Psychiatry*, 6 (1), 7.

Shi, J., Perry, G., Smith, M. A., and Friedland, R. P. (2000). 'Vascular abnormalities: The insidious pathogenesis of Alzheimer's disease', *Neurobiology of Aging*, 21 (2), 357–361.

Shively, S., Scher, A. I., Perl, D. P., and Diaz-Arrastia, R. (2012). 'Dementia resulting from traumatic brain injury: What is the pathology?', *Archives of Neurology*, 69 (10), 1245–1251.

Smebye, K. L., Kirkevold, M., and Engedal, K. (2015). 'Ethical dilemmas concerning autonomy when persons with dementia wish to live at home: A qualitative, hermeneutic study', *BMC Health Services Research*, 16 (1), 21.

SNDS. (2013–2016). *Scotland's national dementia strategy*. Edinburgh: The Scottish Government, <https://www2.gov.scot/Resource/0042/00423472.pdf>, accessed 8 April 2020.

Snowden, J. S., Bathgate, D., Varma, A., Blackshaw, A., Gibbons, Z. C., and Neary, D. (2001). Distinct behavioural profiles in frontotemporal dementia and semantic dementia. *Journal of Neurology, Neurosurgery & Psychiatry*, 70 (3), 323–332.

Spector, A., Hebditch, M., Stoner, C. R., and Gibbor, L. (2016). 'A biopsychosocial vignette for case conceptualization in dementia (VIG-Dem): Development and pilot study', *International Psychogeriatrics*, 28 (9), 1471–1480.

Steeman, E., De Casterlé, B. D., Godderis, J., and Grypdonck, M. (2006). 'Living with early-stage dementia: A review of qualitative studies', *Journal of Advanced Nursing*, 54 (6), 722–738.

Stephan, B., and Brayne, C. (2008). 'Prevalence and projections of dementia'. *Excellence in Dementia Care: Research into Practice*, 9–34.

Stern, Y. (2009). 'Cognitive reserve', *Neuropsychologia*, 47 (10), 2015–2028.

Stokes, G. (2011). 'Psychosocial interventions in care homes'. In T. Dening and A. Milne (eds), *Mental health and care homes*, 205–219. Oxford: Oxford University Press.

Sussman, T., and Regehr, C. (2009). 'The influence of community-based services on the burden of spouses caring for their partners with dementia', *Health & Social Work*, 34 (1), 29–39.

Svendsen, M. N., Navne, L. E., Gjødsbøl, I. M., and Dam, M. S. (2018). 'A life worth living: Temporality, care, and personhood in the Danish welfare state', *American Ethnologist*, 45 (1), 20–33.

Taft, L. B., Fazio, S., Seman, D., and Stansell, J. (1997). 'A psychosocial model of dementia care: Theoretical and empirical support', *Archives of Psychiatric Nursing*, 11 (1), 13–20.

Tan B., Fox S., Kruger C., Lynch M., Shanagher D., and Timmons S (2019). 'Investigating the healthcare utilisation and other support needs of people with young-onset dementia', *Maturitas*, 122, 31–34.

Taylor, J. L., Lindsay, W. R., and Willner, P. (2008). 'CBT for people with intellectual disabilities: Emerging evidence, cognitive ability and IQ effects', *Behavioural and Cognitive Psychotherapy*, 36 (6), 723–733.

Teahan, Á., Lafferty, A., McAuliffe, E., Phelan, A., O'Sullivan, L., O'Shea, D., and Fealy, G. (2018). 'Resilience in family caregiving for people with dementia: A systematic review', *International journal of Geriatric Psychiatry*, 33 (12), 1582–1595.

Teahan, Á., Lafferty, A., Cullinan, J., Fealy, G. and O'Shea, E. (2020). 'An analysis of carer burden among family carers of people with and without dementia in Ireland', *International Psychogeriatrics*, 1–12.

The Institute of Public Health in Ireland (2018). *Improving home care services in Ireland: An overview of the findings of the Department of Health's Public Consultation*. Dublin: Institute of Public Health, Ireland.

Tilse, C., Wilson, J., and Setterland, D. (eds) (2009). 'Personhood, financial decision-making and dementia'. In D. O'Connor and B. Purves (eds), *Decision-making, personhood and dementia: Exploring the interface*, 133–143. London: Jessica Kingsley Publishers.

Timonen, V. (2009). 'Toward an integrative theory of care: Formal and informal intersections'. In J. A. Mancini and K. A. Roberto (eds), *Pathways of human development: Explorations of change*, 307–326. Lexington Books/Rowman & Littlefield.

Travers, C., Lie, D., and Martin Khan, M. (2015). 'Dementia and the population health approach: Promise, pitfalls and progress. An Australian perspective', *Reviews in Clinical Gerontology*, 25, 60–71.

Twigg, J., and Atkin, K. (1994). *Carers perceived: Policy and practice in informal care*. McGraw-Hill Education (UK).

Ungerson, C. (1987). *Policy is personal: Sex, gender and informal care*. Tavistock. ISBN: 0422785008

van den Dungen, P., van Kuijk, L., van Marwijk, H., van der Wouden, J., van Charante, E. M., van der Horst, H., and van Hout, H. (2014). 'Preferences regarding disclosure of a diagnosis of dementia: A systematic review', *International Psychogeriatrics*, 26 (10), 1603–1618.

Verbakel, E., Tamlagsrønning, S., Winstone, L., Fjær, E. L., and Eikemo, T. A. (2017). 'Informal care in Europe: Findings from the European Social Survey (2014) special module on the social determinants of health', *The European Journal of Public Health*, 27 (suppl_1), 90–95.

Verbeek, H. (2011). *Redesigning dementia care: An evaluation of small-scale, homelike care environments* (PhD thesis), Maastricht University, The Netherlands.

Verbeek, H., van Rossum, E., Zwakhalen, S. M., Kempen, G. I., and Hamers, J. P. (2009). 'Small, homelike care environments for older people with dementia: A literature review', *International Psychogeriatrics*, 21 (02), 252–264.

Verbeek, H., Zwakhalen, S. M., Schols, J. M., and Hamers, J. P. (2013). 'Keys to successfully embedding scientific research in nursing homes: A win-win perspective', *Journal of the American Medical Directors Association*, 14 (12), 855–857.

Vernooij-Dassen, M., Moniz-Cook, E., Verhey, F., Chattat, R., Woods, B., Meiland, F., Franco, M., Holmerova, I., Orrell, M., and de Vugt, M. (2019). 'Bridging the divide between biomedical and psychosocial approaches in dementia research: The 2019 INTERDEM Manifesto', *Aging & Mental Health*, 1–7.

Viña, J., and Lloret, A. (2010). 'Why women have more Alzheimer's disease than men: Gender and mitochondrial toxicity of amyloid-β peptide', *Journal of Alzheimer's Disease*, 20 (s2), S527–S533.

Vogt, H., Ulvestad, E., Eriksen, T. E., and Getz, L. (2014). 'Getting personal: Can systems medicine integrate scientific and humanistic conceptions of the patient?', *Journal of Evaluation in Clinical Practice*, 20 (6), 942–952.

von Kutzleben, M., Schmid, W., Halek, M., Holle, B., and Bartholomeyczik, S. (2012). 'Community-dwelling persons with dementia: What do they need? What do they demand? What do they do? A systematic review on the subjective experiences of persons with dementia', *Aging & Mental Health*, 16 (3), 378–390.

Walsh, S., Pertl, M., Gillespie, P., Lawlor, B., Brennan, S., & O'Shea, E. (2019). 'Factors influencing the cost of care and admission to long-term care for people with dementia in Ireland', *Aging & Mental Health*, 1–9.

Watts, S., Cheston, R., Moniz-Cook, E., Burley, C., and Guss, R. (2013). 'Post-diagnostic support for people living with dementia', *Clinical Psychology in the Early Stage Dementia Care Pathway*, 1–13.

Welsh, S., Hassiotis, A., O'Mahoney, G., and Deahl, M. (2003). 'Big brother is watching you--the ethical implications of electronic surveillance measures in the elderly with dementia and in adults with learning difficulties', *Aging & Mental Health*, 7 (5), 372–375.

WHO. (2012). *Dementia: A public health priority.* World Health Organisation (WHO). ISBN: 978 92 4 156445 8, <https://www.who.int/mental_health/publications/dementia_report_2012/en/>, accessed 8 April 2020.

WHO. (2017). *Global action plan on the public health response to dementia 2017–2025.* World Health Organisation (WHO), ISBN 978-92-4-151348-7, <https://www.who.int/mental_health/neurology/dementia/action_plan_2017_2025/en/>, accessed 8 April 2020.

WHO. (2019). 'Risk reduction of cognitive decline and dementia: World Health Organization', WHO guidelines. In *Risk reduction of cognitive decline and dementia: WHO guidelines*, 401–401.

Willemse, B. M., Smit, D., de Lange, J., and Pot, A. M. (2011). 'Nursing home care for people with dementia and residents' quality of life, quality of care and staff well-being: Design of the Living Arrangements for people with Dementia (LAD)-study', *BMC Geriatrics*, 11 (1), 11.

Wimo, A., Wallin, J. O., Lundgren, K., Rönnbäck, E., Asplund, K., Mattsson, B., and Krakau, I. (1991). 'Group living, an alternative for dementia patients. A cost analysis', *International Journal of Geriatric Psychiatry*, 6 (1), 21–29.

Winblad, B., Amouyel, P., Andrieu, S., Ballard, C., Brayne, C., Brodaty, H., Cedazo-Minguez, A., Dubois, B., Edvardsson, D., Feldman, H., Fratiglioni, L., Frisoni, G. B., Gauthier, S., Georges, J., Graff, C., Iqbal, K., Jessen, F., Johansson, G., Jönsson, L., Kivipelto, M., Knapp, M., Mangialasche, F., Melis, R., Nordberg, A., Rikkert, M. O., Qiu, C., Sakmar, T. P., Scheltens, P., Schneider, L. S., Sperling, R., Tjernberg, L. O., Waldemar, G., Wimo, A., and Zetterberg, H. (2016). 'Defeating Alzheimer's disease and other dementias: A priority for European science and society', *The Lancet Neurology*, 15 (5), 455.

Wolfs, C. A., Kessels, A., Severens, J. L., Brouwer, W., de Vugt, M. E., Verhey, F. R., and Dirksen, C. D. (2012). 'Predictive factors for the objective burden of informal care in people with dementia: A systematic review', *Alzheimer Disease & Associated Disorders*, 26 (3), 197–204.

Woods, B., Aguirre, E., Spector, A. E., and Orrell, M. (2012). 'Cognitive stimulation to improve cognitive functioning in people with dementia', *Cochrane Database of Systematic Reviews*, 2.

Woods, R. T., Wills, W., Higginson, I. J., Hobbins, J., and Whitby, M. (2003). 'Support in the community for people with dementia and their carers: A comparative outcome study of specialist mental health service interventions', *International Journal of Geriatric Psychiatry*, 18 (4), 298–307.

Workman, B., Dickson, F., and Green, S. (2010). 'Early dementia: Optimal management in general practice', *Australian Family Physician*, 39 (10), 722.

Wu, Y. T., Fratiglioni, L., Matthews, F. E., Lobo, A., Breteler, M. M., Skoog, I., and Brayne, C. (2016). 'Dementia in western Europe: Epidemiological evidence and implications for policy making', *The Lancet Neurology*, 15 (1), 116–124.

Zarit, S. H., and Zarit, J. M. (2007). Mental disorders in older adults. *Family Caregiving*.

Zarit, S. H., Reever, K. E., and Bach-Peterson, J. (1980). 'Relatives of the impaired elderly: Correlates of feelings of burden', *The Gerontologist*, 20 (6), 649–655.

Zigante, V. (2018). 'Informal care in Europe', *Exploring Formalisation, Availability and Quality, EC*.

Notes on Contributors

SUZANNE CAHILL

Professor Suzanne Cahill was born in Dublin and is a graduate of University College Dublin and a post-graduate of Stockholm University and the University of Queensland Australia. Most of her academic career has been spent teaching, researching and campaigning for the rights of people living with dementia and their family caregivers. She is recognized nationally and internationally as a commentator and expert on dementia matters and she has published a large numbers of scientific articles, book chapters and reports on ageing and dementia. She is author of the book titled: 'Dementia and Human Rights' and was lead author on the research report- 'Creating Excellence in Dementia Care' that underpinned Ireland's first national Dementia Strategy. She is currently an Adjunct Professor of Social Work and Social Policy at Trinity College Dublin. She also holds an honorary professorship in Dementia Care at the Centre for Economic and Social Research on Dementia in NUI Galway and is an affiliated Professor in Health and Welfare at the Institute of Gerontology in Jönkoping University Sweden.

KATHY RYAN

Kathy Ryan was diagnosed with young-onset Alzheimer's disease in January 2014 at the age of 53. The pathway she had to this diagnosis and its disclosure was not straightforward. She is the Chairperson of the Irish Dementia Working Group and a member of the Dementia Research Advisory Team, both of which are supported by The Alzheimer Society of Ireland (ASI). Kathy is a strong and powerful self-advocate for dementia and her advocacy work currently brings her all over Ireland where she is committed to upskilling the public about dementia and lobbying for improved dementia services and supports. Kathy sits on a number of National Steering Groups, speaks at conferences where she educates many health service professionals about the lived experience of dementia. Kathy has also participated in a large number of research projects across Ireland and more recently has contributed to projects in a patient and public involvement (PPI) capacity. As a member of the ASI's Dementia Research Advisory Team, Kathy regularly participates in capacity-building workshops centred on PPI. In this role she feels empowered to be an effective PPI contributor in research studies.

Index

A

activities 8, 35, 40, 42, 59, 62, 66, 94, 98–100, 104, 109
　activity of daily living 10, 42, 59, 63, 72
Alzheimer Europe (AE) 3, 5, 32, 38, 43, 44, 82, 98
Alzheimer Society of Ireland (ASI) 14, 15, 22, 41, 45, 47, 48, 52, 53, 70, 108, 113
Alzheimer's disease 1, 2, 4, 5, 7, 10, 11, 17, 19, 21, 23, 48–50, 53, 75, 110, 111
Alzheimer's disease dementia (AD dementia) 1, 5, 10, 11
Alzheimer's Disease International (ADI) 3, 7, 27, 33, 34, 42, 86, 88
Assisted Decision-Making Capacity Act (ADMCA) 54, 83–86, 89
assisted living facilities 105
Atlantic Philanthropies 12, 16, 17, 29, 35, 36, 107
autonomy 23, 34, 37, 61, 62, 75, 77, 78, 79, 81–89, 98, 102, 109, 112

B

behavioural and psychological symptoms of dementia 21, 63
behaviours that challenge 59, 63, 64, 66, 72, 96, 112
biopsychosocial 23, 24, 28, 29, 79, 80

C

capacity
　legal 28, 82
　mental 82, 84, 85, 86, 87, 88, 112

care
　home care services 13, 68, 73, 87, 92, 100, 105, 111, 114
　long-term 14, 78, 91–94, 97–100, 102, 103, 105, 106
　new culture 102
　old culture 80 *see* Kitwood
　staff 24, 36, 100, 103, 105, 107, 108, 111
caregiver burden 43, 57, 65, 71, 73, 96
　objective 65, 66
　subjective 65, 66
caregiver stress 66
　stress-coping models 57, 65, 66
caregivers
　adult children 60, 61, 71, 73
　family 38, 41, 43, 44, 58, 60, 65, 67, 68, 71, 72, 85, 109, 111, 112
　formal 58, 75, 109, 114
　informal 15, 57, 58–61, 63, 65–71, 73, 105, 111, 114
　spouse 7, 57, 60, 61, 69, 71, 72, 73, 96
caregiving tasks
　advanced 64
　early 61, 62
　moderate 62, 63
carer's
　allowance 58, 69, 71
　benefit 69
　leave act 69
　support grant 69
citizenship 24, 25, 28, 29, 108, 114
　everyday 25
　social 24
cognitive rehabilitation (CR) 34, 40, 41–42, 46, 114
cognitive reserve 8–9
cognitive stimulation therapy (CST) 40, 42–43, 46, 104, 114

community 13, 15, 29, 36, 38, 58, 67, 87, 100, 101, 108
  care/based services 13, 38, 41, 70, 76, 92, 100
  living/dwelling 22, 41, 44, 67, 70, 108
complexities 39
  dementia 39, 110–111
  family caregiving 111–112
conflicting policy agendas 59
  see also policy
continuum of care 73, 97–99, 106
Convention on the Rights of Persons with Disability (CRPD) 26, 81, 83, 113
cost(s) 3, 4, 7, 12, 15, 17, 52, 58, 66, 68, 93, 94, 100, 104

D

decision-making 34, 35, 39, 44, 45, 62, 75, 77, 79, 81–89, 112
  substitute 82, 85
  supportive 82, 85
dementia advisors 39, 44, 45, 53
dementia advisors/advisory services 22, 41, 45
Dementia Services Information and Development Centre (DSIDC) 15, 16, 99
dementia stages
  advanced/severe 2, 10, 38, 64, 79, 80, 100
  early 2, 34, 41, 61, 62, 86
  moderate 2, 10, 38, 62, 100
dementia sub-types
  Alzheimer's disease 4–5
  dementia with Lewy body 6
  frontotemporal 6
  vascular dementia 6
Denmark 98

diagnosis 31–36
  benefits 32, 33, 45
  early 31–33, 45, 54
  timely 31–33, 54, 86, 111
diagnostic services 31, 36, 46, 97, 108, 113
  post-diagnostic services 25, 31, 33, 35, 37, 38–45, 46, 97, 108
disclosure 31, 36, 37, 45, 86, 113
drugs/medications 9, 10, 11, 34, 36, 42, 48–51, 62, 63, 81, 104

E

enduring power of attorney (EPA) 34, 62, 85, 86
environment(s) 63, 86–88, 97, 98, 100, 102, 103, 105, 108, 111
  built/physical 21, 101, 102
  psycho-social 22, 78, 91, 101

F

family caregivers 38, 41, 43, 44, 58, 60, 65, 67, 68, 71, 72, 85, 109, 111, 112
France 11, 44, 107, 114
functional 20, 23, 27, 41, 83, 95, 96
future directions 112–113

G

general practitioners (GP) 28, 34, 35–37, 45, 47–49, 51, 108, 111, 113
global action plan (WHO) 27, 86

H

health 1, 2, 8, 9, 15, 17, 19, 20, 24, 26–28, 34, 36, 41, 44, 47, 51, 64, 65, 66, 68, 70, 71, 72, 77, 78, 84, 85, 86, 96, 97, 100, 108, 110, 114
Health Act 93

health care assistant 82
health care professional/health service professionals 12, 29, 44, 72, 82, 84, 108, 111
health care representative (HCR) 85, 86
Health Information Quality Authority (HIQA) 93
Health Services Executive (HSE) 12, 14, 22, 28, 35, 40, 45, 92, 93, 94, 99
home care 13, 68, 69, 92, 112
    home care packages 70, 92
    intensive home care packages 13, 70, 87, 108
    support/services/scheme 13, 72, 73, 87, 92, 100, 105, 106, 111, 112, 114
human rights 25, 26, 28, 88, 104

I

impairments 2, 21, 22, 26, 28, 72, 78
    cognitive 5, 10, 13, 26, 34, 37, 38, 49, 66, 70, 75, 83, 87, 89, 95
    functional 27, 95, 96
incidence rates 1, 11, 12, 17, 113
independence 23, 33, 62, 75, 102, 112
Ireland 31, 34, 35, 36, 37, 38, 40, 41, 42, 43, 44, 45, 46, 57, 58, 66, 67, 68, 69, 70, 71, 76, 82, 83, 85, 87, 91, 92, 93, 95, 96, 98, 99, 100, 101, 104, 105, 107, 108, 109, 113, 114
    aging 11, 28, 92, 93, 94
    dementia 1, 11–17, 19, 22, 29, 53, 54, 86, 95, 98, 99, 104, 105, 107, 108, 109, 110 111, 112, 114
    dementia policy 17
Irish
    Government 13, 15, 16, 35, 68
    research/studies 37, 40, 73
    working group 15, 113

K

Khan, R. L.
    biomedical model 77
    excess disability 78
    hierarchical structures 78
    psycho-social-biological 78
    senility 18, 78
Kitwood, T.
    definition of personhood 79
    good dementia care 80
    holistic approach to dementia 23
    old culture of care 80
    preserving personhood 88
    re-conceptualizing dementia 81
    theory of dementia and personhood 80

L

language 2, 4, 5, 6, 20, 31, 52, 64, 76
    speech and language therapists 23, 104
legislation 13, 68, 69, 85, 89, 98, 112
loneliness 107
long term care, *see* care

M

media 53
medications *see* drugs/medications
memory clinic 36, 37, 42, 43, 48, 49, 113, 114
mild cognitive impairment (MCI) 5, 10, 11, 17, 32
models of dementia
    biomedical 5, 19–21, 23, 28, 29, 77, 80, 100
    biopsychosocial 23–24, 29
    citizenship 24–25, 28
    human rights 25–26, 28
    social 21–23, 26, 28

mortality 111
multidisciplinary 29
multisensory 102

N

National Dementia Office (NDO) 12, 20, 28, 36, 40, 42–44, 46, 108
National Dementia Strategy (NDS) 12–14, 16, 26, 28, 29, 32, 35, 40, 45, 70, 86, 107, 108, 113
Netherlands 44, 98, 101
Norway 99
nursing home care 72, 93, 96, 103–105, 111
nursing homes 14, 58, 87, 92–105, 107

O

old culture of care 80
outdoors/environment 103

P

personalized 22, 62, 64, 70, 73, 102, 103, 104, 111, 114
personhood 24, 29, 37, 62, 70, 75, 77, 78, 79–83, 85, 86, 87, 88, 89, 98, 102, 108, 109, 114
policy 11, 17, 19, 59, 76, 89, 91, 97, 99, 102, 104, 105, 109, 110, 112, 113
    government 13, 16, 35, 68, 73, 92
    plans 4, 12, 39, 107, 114
    prevention 26
    public 27
    social care 1, 17
policy makers 13, 31, 38, 100
preferences 32, 81, 83, 105
prevalence rates 1, 3, 6, 7, 11, 12, 17, 95, 105, 113
psychosocial educational intervention (PEI) 40, 43, 44

public health 19, 27, 86
public policy 27

R

reablement 23
rehabilitation 29, 41, 42
relational autonomy 83
research 11, 16, 19–21, 27, 35, 37, 40, 49, 53, 55, 71, 81, 96, 101, 107, 108, 109, 110, 112, 113
    biomedical research 5, 21
    future/further research 11, 97
    health service research 109
    longitudinal research 101
    quantitative research 20, 96
    research perspective 20
    research review 16
residential care 13, 24, 38, 57, 68, 70, 71, 72, 76, 77–78, 87, 88, 91–101, 103–106, 112
rights 24, 25–26, 28, 82, 86, 87, 88, 89, 112
risk factors 1, 2, 7, 8, 14, 17, 27
Rochford-Brennan, H. 113

S

Sabat, R. 20
    biomedical model 20–21
    biopsychosocial model 23, 79
    excess disabilities 22
    mental capacity 82
    negative positioning 76
Scotland/Scottish 39, 44
senility 4, 5, 9, 76–78
services
    dementia care 12, 16, 17, 22, 23, 39, 77, 78, 91, 106, 108, 113, 114
    health care 77, 100
    palliative care 3, 97
    social care 15, 20, 26, 27, 29, 37, 58

special care units 96, 99, 105
stigma/stigmatizing/de-stigmatizing 14, 26, 27, 33, 55, 76, 108
Sweden/Swedish 11, 98, 99

T

technology 35
training 35, 43, 44, 71, 88, 103, 108, 110, 113
treatment(s)
    drugs/pharmacological 3, 10, 11, 14, 19, 20, 21, 28, 34, 37, 39, 104
    non-drugs/non-pharmacological/psychosocial 3, 14, 39, 94

U

understandings/misunderstandings 4, 14, 75, 79, 81

United Kingdom (UK) 42, 43, 79, 95, 107, 114
United Nations Convention on the Rights of Persons with Disabilities, *see* Convention on the Rights of Persons with Disability
United States of America (USA) 65, 97, 98, 107

W

will and preference 84, 85
World Health Organization (WHO) 27, 98

Y

young-onset dementia 4, 5, 7, 13, 37, 38, 46, 54, 113

www.ingramcontent.com/pod-product-compliance
Ingram Content Group UK Ltd.
Pitfield, Milton Keynes, MK11 3LW, UK
UKHW021834140426
5217IPUK00021B/1437